The 12-Lead ECG

IN ACUTE CORONARY SYNDROMES

5TH EDITION

The 12-Lead ECG

IN ACUTE CORONARY SYNDROMES

Barbara Aehlert, MSEd, BSPA, RN
President, Southwest EMS Education, Inc.

Tim Phalen
President, ECG Solutions, Inc.

ELSEVIER

Elsevier
3251 Riverport Lane
St. Louis, Missouri 63043

THE 12-LEAD ECG IN ACUTE CORONARY SYNDROMES, FIFTH EDITION   ISBN: 978-0-443-12208-8

Previous edition copyrighted 2019, 2012, 2006, 1996.

Content Strategist: Kelly Skelton
Content Development Specialist: Deborah Poulson
Publishing Services Manager: Deepthi Unni
Senior Project Manager: Kamatchi Madhavan
Senior Book Designer: Amy Buxton

Printed in India

Last digit is the print number: 9   8   7   6   5   4   3   2   1

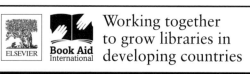

Preface

The challenge in providing a simplified method of 12-lead electrocardiogram (ECG) acquisition and infarct recognition lies in determining the information essential for the effective identification and treatment of acute coronary syndromes. If a text provides too much information, you are quickly overwhelmed. If it supplies inadequate information, it is of little benefit to your clinical practice. In writing this book, we attempted to walk that fine line and avoid both outcomes.

We have assumed that the reader has successfully completed an introductory ECG recognition course before undertaking 12-lead ECG interpretation. As a result, we have chosen to provide only a brief review of waveform identification and measurement, and rate and rhythm determination. We assume that the reader is proficient in basic dysrhythmia recognition.

We know that the transition from interpreting ECGs in a textbook to using 12-lead ECG interpretive skills in clinical practice is a big step. To help you make the leap, we present information in an easy-to-understand format. Using tables, illustrations, and a large number of practice 12-lead ECGs, you will learn to recognize ST-elevation myocardial infarction (STEMI), non–ST-elevation myocardial infarction (NSTEMI), and common ST-elevation variants.

With this edition, we feel it is important to recognize the increasing presence of nonphysician practitioners (NPPs)—that is, physician assistants and advanced-practice nurses in prehospital and hospital settings. NPPs play a vital role in caring for patients with ischemic heart disease, both during and after an acute ischemic event. With this in mind, and where appropriate, the word "physician" has been changed to "provider" throughout this text.

We have made every effort to offer information consistent with current literature; however, we encourage you to learn and follow local protocols as defined by your medical advisors. We hope this text gives you a practical jump-start toward infarct recognition, convinces you that 12-leads do not have to be intimidating, and encourages you to learn even more advanced electrocardiography.

Barbara Aehlert
Tim Phalen

Acknowledgments

Our thanks to the manuscript reviewer, who provided insightful comments and suggestions. A special thanks to Deborah Poulson for her assistance with this project, and to Dr. Greg Lachar, Andrew Baird, Andrea Lowrey, Paul Honeywell, and Jay Wood for providing many of the 12-lead ECGs used in this text.

Barbara Aehlert
Tim Phalen

About the Authors

Barbara Aehlert has been a registered nurse for more than 40 years, with clinical experience in medical/surgical nursing, critical care nursing, prehospital education, and nursing education.

Since 1994, Tim Phalen has led ECG workshops for more than 75,000 participants in a dozen countries. Before he became a full-time speaker, Tim was a paramedic for 14 years. He began integrating 12-lead ECGs into patient care in the 1980s. Tim feels fortunate to have learned from many great instructors along the way, of whom the most helpful and influential was Dr. Henry Marriott.

Reviewer for the Fifth Edition

Chris Wright, BS, RCIS, EMT-P
Clinical Sales Specialist
Abbott Structural Heart- TAVI
Ann Arbor, Michigan

Contents

Reviewing the Basics

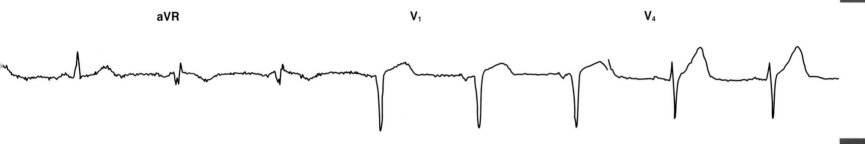

LEARNING OBJECTIVES

After reading this chapter, you should be able to:

1. Identify and describe the heart's layers, chambers, valves, and surfaces.
2. Describe the flow of blood through the normal heart and lungs to the systemic circulation.
3. Name the primary branches and areas of the heart supplied by the right and left coronary arteries.
4. Appreciate the variance in normal coronary artery distribution.
5. Describe the normal sequence of electrical conduction through the heart.
6. Define and describe each of the waveforms, segments, complexes, and intervals as they relate to electrical activity in the heart.

KEY TERMS

acute coronary syndromes: Distinct conditions caused by a similar sequence of pathologic events involving abruptly reduced coronary artery blood flow

baseline: Straight line recorded on electrocardiographic graph paper when no electrical activity is detected

biphasic: Waveform that is partly positive and partly negative

complex: Several waveforms

depolarization: Movement of ions across a cell membrane causing the inside of the cell to become more positive; an electrical event expected to result in contraction

interval: A waveform and a segment

ischemia: Decreased supply of oxygenated blood to a body part or organ

isoelectric line: Absence of electrical activity; observed on the electrocardiogram as a straight line

repolarization: Movement of ions across a cell membrane in which the inside of the cell is restored to its negative charge

segment: Line between waveforms; named by the waveform that precedes and follows it

STRUCTURE OF THE HEART

The human heart is a four-chambered muscular organ that is about the size of the individual's fist. It lies between the lungs in the mediastinum. The heart is protected anteriorly by the sternum and ribs and posteriorly by the ribs and vertebral column. About two-thirds of the heart lies to the left of the midline of the sternum.

The anterior surface of the heart is formed by portions of the right atrium and the left and right ventricles (Fig. 1.1). However, because the heart is tilted slightly toward the left in the chest, the right ventricle is the area of the heart that lies most directly behind the sternum. The heart's left side (i.e., left lateral surface) is composed chiefly of the left ventricle. The heart's inferior surface, also called the *diaphragmatic* surface, is formed primarily by the left ventricle with a small portion of the right ventricle.

Heart Chambers and Valves

The heart's two thin-walled upper chambers are the right and left atria, which serve to receive blood. The right and left ventricles comprise the two thicker-walled lower chambers (Fig. 1.2), which are responsible for pumping blood.

The right side of the heart is a low-pressure system (i.e., the pulmonary circuit). The right atrium receives blood from the superior vena cava, the inferior vena cava, and the

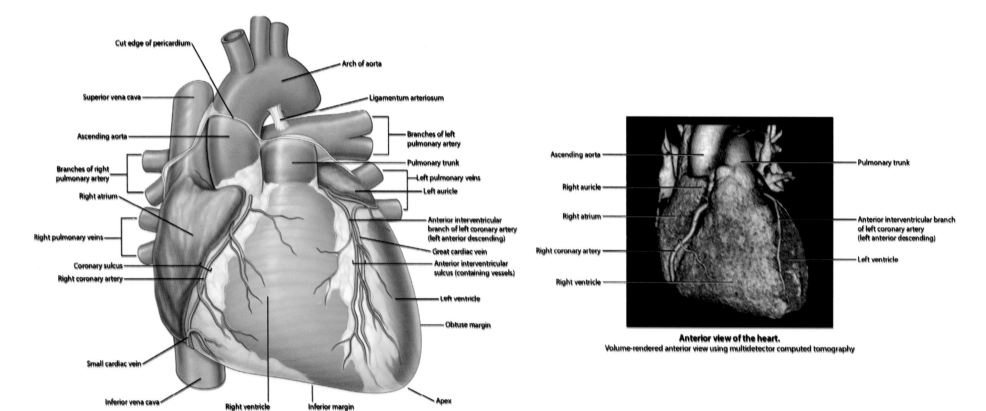

Anterior surface of the heart

Fig. **1.1** The anterior surface of the heart. (From Drake, R., Vogl, A.W., & Mitchell, A.W.M. [2021]. *Gray's atlas of anatomy* [3rd ed.]. Elsevier.)

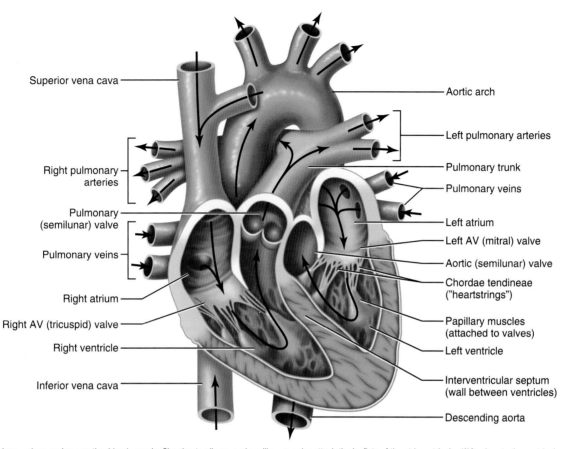

Fig. **1.2** Internal view of the heart showing chambers, valves, and connecting blood vessels. Chordae tendineae and papillary muscles attach the leaflets of the atrioventricular (AV) valves to the ventricular myocardium. Arrows indicate the direction of blood flow. (From Solomon, E. P. [2016]. *Introduction to human anatomy and physiology* [4th ed.]. Saunders.)

coronary sinus. Blood entering the right ventricle flows through the tricuspid valve to the right ventricle. The right ventricle pumps the blood through the pulmonic semilunar (SL) valve to the pulmonary trunk, which divides into the right and left pulmonary arteries. The pulmonary arteries enter the right and left lungs, where the exchange of oxygen and carbon dioxide occurs. Oxygenated blood is returned to the heart's left atrium through four pulmonary veins, two from each lung.

The left side of the heart is a high-pressure pump (i.e., the systemic circuit). The left atrium receives oxygenated blood from four pulmonary veins, two from each lung. Blood flows from the left atrium through the mitral valve to the left ventricle. The left ventricle must overcome a lot of pressure and resistance from the arteries and contract forcefully to pump blood through the aortic SL valve and out to the body.

Consider This

Each ventricle holds about 150 mL of blood when full. They normally eject about half this volume (70 to 80 mL) with each contraction. The stroke volume is the amount of blood ejected from a ventricle with each heartbeat. The ejection fraction is the percentage of blood pumped out of a ventricle with each contraction. The ejection fraction is used as a measure of ventricular function. A normal ejection fraction is between 50% and 65%. A person is said to have impaired ventricular function when the ejection fraction is less than 40%. Patients with a poor ejection fraction may include those with heart failure, severe cardiomyopathy, or myocardial damage from a previous heart attack.

Four one-way valves in the heart ensure the forward flow of blood through the heart's chambers. The tricuspid and mitral valves are atrioventricular (AV) valves that allow blood to flow from the atria into the ventricles when the ventricles are relaxed (ventricular diastole). Chordae tendineae, thin strands of connective tissue, are attached to the underside of the AV valves on one end. On the other end, they are bound to papillary muscles, which are small mounds of myocardium. Papillary muscles project inward from the lower portion of the ventricular walls. The chordae tendineae and papillary muscles serve as anchors. When the ventricles contract and relax, the papillary muscles adjust their tension on the chordae tendineae, preventing them from bulging too far into the atria.

The pulmonic and aortic valves are SL valves that prevent the backflow of blood from the aorta and pulmonary arteries into the left and right ventricles, respectively. Unlike the AV valves, the SL valves are not attached to chordae tendineae. Blood flow through the normal heart and pulmonary circulation is summarized in Box 1.1.

Box **1.1**	**Blood Flow Through the Normal Heart and Pulmonary Circulation**

Blood from the superior and inferior vena cavae and the coronary sinus enters the right atrium → tricuspid valve → right ventricle → pulmonic semilunar valve → pulmonary trunk → right and left pulmonary arteries → pulmonary capillaries (within the lungs) → four pulmonary veins → left atrium → mitral valve → left ventricle → aortic semilunar valve → ascending aorta

Heart Layers

The heart's walls are made up of three tissue layers: the endocardium, myocardium, and epicardium. The endocardium is the innermost layer. It lines the heart's inner chambers, valves, chordae tendineae, and papillary muscles. It is continuous with the innermost layer of the body's arteries, veins, and capillaries. The middle layer, the myocardium, is the thickest. It consists of cardiac muscle cells that contract and relax. The subendocardial area is the innermost half of the myocardium, and the outermost half is the subepicardial area. The outermost layer is the epicardium, also called the *visceral pericardium*. It contains blood and lymph capillaries, nerve fibers, and fat. This layer is enveloped by the pericardial sac, which anchors the heart within the chest.

Coronary Vessels

The work of the heart is vital. To ensure that it has an adequate blood supply, the heart makes sure to provide itself with a fresh supply of oxygenated blood before supplying the rest of the body. This freshly oxygenated blood is provided mainly by the branches of two vessels—the right and left coronary arteries. The openings to these vessels lie just beyond the cusps of the aortic SL valve.

The right and left coronary arteries are found on the heart's epicardial surface. They feed this area first before their branches penetrate the myocardium to supply the subendocardium with blood (Fig. 1.3). The diameter of these "feeder branches" (i.e., collateral circulation) is much narrower.

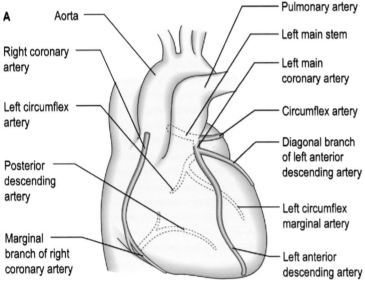
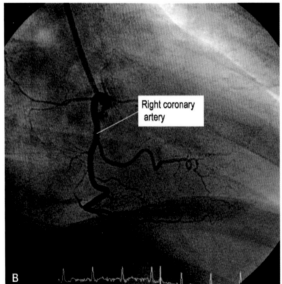
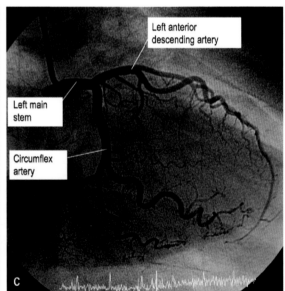

Fig. **1.3** Coronary circulation. (A) Normal coronary arterial anatomy. (B) Angiogram of the dominant right coronary system. (C) Angiogram of the left coronary system from the same patient. (From Feather, A., Randall, D., & Waterhouse, M. [2021]. *Kumar and Clark's clinical medicine* [10th ed.]. Elsevier.)

When a temporary or permanent blockage occurs in a coronary artery, the blood supply to the heart muscle is impaired, and myocardial cells distal to the site of the blockage are starved for oxygen and other nutrients. **Acute coronary syndromes (ACSs)** are a group of conditions caused by an abrupt reduction in coronary artery blood flow. The sequence of events that occurs during an ACS results in conditions that range from myocardial **ischemia** (i.e., unstable angina [UA] pectoris) to death (i.e., necrosis) of the heart muscle (with or without associated ST-segment elevation [STE] on the electrocardiogram [ECG]). An understanding of coronary artery anatomy and the areas of the heart that each vessel supplies can help you predict which coronary artery is blocked and anticipate problems associated with the blockage of that vessel.

Right Coronary Artery

The right coronary artery (RCA) originates from the right side of the aorta. It travels along the groove between the right atrium and right ventricle. Branches of the RCA supply blood to the right atrium, right ventricle, and the inferior and posterior walls of the left ventricle in most individuals.

Left Coronary Artery

The left coronary artery (LCA) originates from the left side of the aorta. The first segment of the LCA is the left main coronary artery, also called the *left main trunk* (see Fig. 1.3). It supplies oxygenated blood to its two primary branches: the left anterior descending (LAD), also called the *anterior interventricular* artery, and the circumflex artery (Cx). These vessels are slightly smaller than the left main coronary artery.

In most people, the LAD travels along the groove between the right and left ventricles, courses along the heart's apex, and ends along the left ventricle's inferior surface. In the remaining individuals, the LAD does not reach the inferior surface. Instead, it stops at or before the heart's apex. The major branches of the LAD are the septal and diagonal arteries. The septal branches of the LAD supply blood to the interventricular septum. The diagonal branches supply the anterior and lateral walls of the left ventricle. The Cx circles around the left side of the heart and supplies blood to the left atrium, part of the left ventricle's lateral wall, and the left ventricle's inferior and posterior surfaces.

Coronary Artery Dominance

The blood supply to the inferior and posterior areas of the left ventricle varies. The coronary artery that forms the posterior descending artery (PDA) is considered the dominant coronary artery. The RCA forms the PDA in about 70% to 80% of people (right dominant); in 5% to 10%, it is formed by the Cx (left dominant). In 10% to 20%, the PDA is supplied by both the Cx and RCA (codominant) (Shahoud et al., 2022). The areas of the heart supplied by the major coronary arteries are shown in Fig. 1.4.

Coronary Veins

Blood that has passed through the myocardial capillaries is drained by branches of the cardiac veins that join the coronary sinus, which lies in the groove (sulcus) that separates the atria from the ventricles. The coronary sinus drains into the right atrium.

CARDIAC CYCLE

The cardiac cycle has two phases for each heart chamber: systole and diastole. Systole is the period during which the chamber contracts and blood is ejected. Diastole is the period of relaxation during which the chambers are allowed to fill. The myocardium receives its fresh supply of oxygenated blood from the coronary arteries during ventricular diastole. The cardiac cycle depends on the cardiac muscle's ability to contract and on the condition of the heart's conduction system. The heart's efficiency as a pump may be affected by abnormalities of the cardiac muscle, the valves, or the conduction system.

During the cardiac cycle, the pressure within each chamber of the heart rises in systole and falls in diastole. The heart's valves ensure that blood flows in the proper direction. Blood flows from one heart chamber to another from higher to lower pressure. These pressure relationships depend on the careful timing of contractions. The heart's conduction system provides the necessary timing of events between atrial and ventricular systole.

ELECTROPHYSIOLOGY REVIEW

Human body fluids contain electrolytes, which are elements or compounds that break into charged particles (i.e., ions) when melted or dissolved in water or another solvent. Differences in the composition of ions between the intracellular and extracellular fluid compartments are essential for normal body function, including the activity of the heart. Body fluids that contain electrolytes conduct an electric current. Electrolytes move about in body fluids and carry a charge.

Potential energy (i.e., voltage) exists because of the imbalance of charged particles across the membranes of cells. This imbalance makes the cells excitable. The membrane potential is the voltage (i.e., the difference in electrical charges) across the cell membrane. The energy the cells expend to move electrolytes across the cell membrane creates a flow of current, expressed in volts. Voltage appears on an ECG as spikes or waveforms.

Depolarization

When a cell is at rest (i.e., polarized), the inside of the cell is more negative than the outside. When stimulated, the cell membrane becomes permeable to sodium (Na^+) and potassium (K^+), allowing the passage of electrolytes after it is open. Na^+ rushes into the cell through Na^+ channels, causing the inside of the cell to become more positive

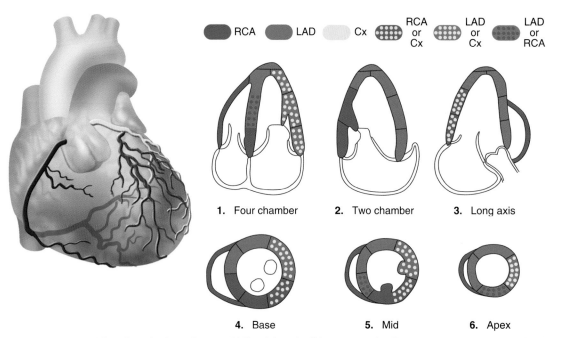

1. Four chamber **2.** Two chamber **3.** Long axis

4. Base **5.** Mid **6.** Apex

Fig. **1.4** Typical myocardial segments supplied by the right coronary artery (RCA), left anterior descending artery (LAD), and circumflex (Cx) coronary arteries. The coronary anatomy is shown on the left, with the corresponding wall segments in standard echocardiographic views on the right. The arterial distribution varies between patients. Some segments have variable coronary perfusion, as indicated by the hatched regions. (From Lang, R. M., Bierig, M., Devereux, R. B., Flachskampf, F. A., Foster, E., Pellikka, P. A., Picard, M. H., Roman, M. J., Seward, J., Shanewise, J. S., Solomon, S. D., Spencer, K. T., Sutton, M. S., Stewart, W. J.; Chamber Quantification Writing Group; American Society of Echocardiography's Guidelines and Standards Committee; European Association of Echocardiography [2005]. Recommendations for Chamber Quantification: A report from the American Society of Echocardiography's Guidelines and Standards Committee and the Chamber Quantification Writing Group, developed in conjunction with the European Association of Echocardiography, a branch of the European Society of Cardiology. *Journal of the American Society of Echocardiography, 18*[12], 1440–1463.)

relative to the outside. The movement of charged particles across a cell membrane that causes the inside of the cell to become positive is called **depolarization**. A waveform is then recorded on the ECG. Depolarization proceeds from the endocardium to the epicardium.

Consider This

Depolarization is an *electrical* event that must occur before the heart can contract and pump blood, which is a *mechanical* event.

An impulse normally begins in the pacemaker cells found in the heart's sinoatrial (SA) node. Then, a chain reaction occurs from cell to cell in the heart's electrical conduction system until all the cells have been stimulated and depolarized. Eventually, the impulse is spread from the pacemaker cells to the working myocardial cells, which contract when stimulated.

Consider This

The ability of cardiac pacemaker cells to create an electrical impulse without being stimulated by another source, such as a nerve, is called *automaticity*. Increased blood concentrations of calcium (Ca^{++}) increase automaticity. Conversely, decreased K^+ concentrations in the blood decrease automaticity.

Repolarization

After the cell depolarizes, it quickly begins to recover and restore its electrical charges to normal. The movement of charged particles across a cell membrane in which the inside of the cell is restored to its negative charge is called **repolarization**. The cell membrane stops the flow of Na^+ into the cell and allows K^+ to leave it. As a result, negatively charged particles are left inside the cell, the cell returns to its resting state, and the contractile proteins in the working myocardial cells separate (i.e., relax). Repolarization proceeds from the epicardium to the endocardium.

Consider This

When the atria are stimulated, a P wave is recorded on the ECG; thus the P wave represents atrial depolarization. When the ventricles are stimulated, a QRS complex is recorded on the ECG; thus the QRS complex represents ventricular depolarization. The ST segment and T wave represent ventricular repolarization. A waveform representing atrial repolarization is usually not seen on the ECG because it is small and buried in the QRS complex.

The Cardiac Action Potential

The action potential of a cardiac cell reflects the rapid sequence of voltage changes across the cell membrane during the electrical cardiac cycle. The action potential configuration varies depending on the cardiac cell's location, size, and function.

CONDUCTION SYSTEM

The heart's conduction system is a collection of specialized pacemaker cells that are arranged in a system of interconnected pathways (Fig. 1.5). The normal heartbeat is the result of an electrical impulse that begins in the SA node, which is specialized conducting tissue located in the upper posterior part of the right atrium where the superior vena cava and the right atrium meet. As the impulse leaves the SA node, a chain reaction occurs from cell to cell in the heart's electrical conduction system until all the cells have been stimulated and depolarized. The conduction system is summarized in Table 1.1.

Secondary Pacemakers

Areas of the heart other than the SA node can initiate beats (i.e., intrinsic automaticity) and assume pacemaker responsibility under special circumstances. The terms *secondary*, *subsidiary*, *latent*, or *ectopic* refer to sites other than the SA node that can assume pacemaking responsibility. Secondary pacemaker sites include the cells of the AV junction and Purkinje fibers, although their intrinsic rates are slower than that of the SA node. A secondary pacemaker is normally prevented from discharging because of the dominance of the SA node's rapidly firing pacemaker cells. A secondary site may assume pacemaker responsibility in the following circumstances: (1) the SA node fires too slowly because of vagal stimulation or suppression by medications; (2) the SA node fails to generate an impulse because of disease or suppression by medications; (3) the SA node action

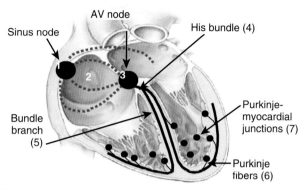

Fig. **1.5** The cardiac action potential originates in the sinoatrial (SA) node (1), continues in the atrial wall (2), and is delayed in the atrioventricular (AV) node (3). Conduction within the ventricles is initially rapid within the rapid conduction system: His bundle (4), right and left bundle branches (5), and Purkinje fibers (6). Next, the impulse is transferred from the rapid conduction system to the working myocardium in the Purkinje-myocardial junctions (7) located in the endocardium. Finally, the impulse is conducted from the endocardium to the epicardium within the slowly conducting working myocardium. (From Ellenbogen, K. A., Wilkoff, B. L., Kay, G. N., Lau, C. P., & Auricchio, A. [2017]. *Clinical cardiac pacing, defibrillation and resynchronization therapy* [5th ed.]. Elsevier.)

TABLE 1.1	Summary of the Conduction System
Structure	**Function**
SA node	• Primary pacemaker; intrinsic pacemaker rate: 60 to 100 beats/min • Initiates impulse that is normally conducted throughout the left and right atria • Supplied by a branch of the RCA in about 60% of individuals
AV node	• Receives impulse from SA node and delays relay of the impulse to the bundle of His, allowing time for ventricular filling before the onset of ventricular contraction
Bundle of His (AV bundle)	• Receives impulse from AV node and relays it to right and left bundle branches • AV node and bundle of His make up the AV junction, which has an intrinsic pacemaker rate of 40 to 60 beats/min • Supplied by a branch of the RCA in 85% to 90% of individuals
Right and left bundle branches	• Receives impulse from bundle of His and relays it to Purkinje fibers
Purkinje fibers	• Receives impulse from bundle branches and relays it to ventricular myocardium • Intrinsic pacemaker rate: 20 to 40 beats/min

AV, Atrioventricular; *RCA*, right coronary artery; *SA*, sinoatrial.

potential is blocked because of disease in conducting pathways, failing to activate the surrounding atrial myocardium; or (4) the firing rate of the ectopic site becomes faster than that of the SA node.

Although secondary pacemakers supply a safety mechanism in the event of SA node failure, these sites can be problematic if they fire while the SA node is still functioning. For example, secondary sites may cause early (i.e., premature) beats or sustained rhythm disturbances.

WAVEFORMS, COMPLEXES, SEGMENTS, AND INTERVALS

ECG paper records the speed and magnitude of the heart's electrical impulses. This graph paper consists of small and large boxes measured in millimeters. The smallest boxes are 1 mm wide and 1 mm high (Fig. 1.6). Each large box, which is the width of five small

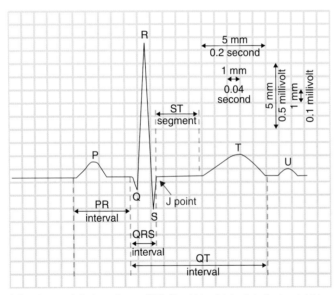

Fig. **1.6** Inscription of a normal electrocardiogram (ECG). Sinoatrial nodal depolarization is not visible on the surface ECG; the P wave corresponds to atrial muscle depolarization. The PR interval represents conduction through the atrial muscle, atrioventricular node, and His-Purkinje system. The QRS complex reflects ventricular muscle depolarization. Ventricular repolarization is represented by the ST segment and T wave (and U wave, if present). The J point lies at the junction of the end of the QRS complex and the beginning of the ST segment. The QT interval is measured from the onset of the QRS to the end of the T wave. Note the gridlines. On the horizontal axis, each 1-mm line ("small" box) denotes 0.04 second (40 msec); a "big" box denotes 0.20 second (200 msec). On the vertical axis, 1 mm (small box) corresponds to 0.1 mV; therefore, 10 mm (two big boxes) denotes 1 mV. (From Goldman, L., & Schafer, A. I. [2020]. *Goldman-Cecil medicine* [26th ed.]. Elsevier.)

boxes, represents 0.20 second. The horizontal axis of the paper corresponds to time. Time is used to measure the interval between or duration of specific cardiac events, which is stated in seconds.

Consider This

When reviewing a 12-lead ECG, intervals and duration are usually expressed in milliseconds (msec). There are 1000 msec in 1 second. Move the decimal point three places to the right when converting from seconds to milliseconds.

The rate at which ECG paper goes through the printer is adjustable and is designated on the 12-lead ECG printout. The standard paper speed is 25 mm/second. At this speed, each 1-mm box represents 0.04 second (40 msec), and each 5-mm gridline, a large box, represents 0.20 second (200 msec). The rate at which ECG paper goes through the printer is adjustable. A faster paper speed makes the rhythm appear slower and the QRS complex wider. Thus in cases of rapid heart rates, a faster paper speed makes it easier to see the waveforms and analyze the rhythm. A slower paper speed makes the rhythm appear faster and the QRS narrower.

The vertical axis of the graph paper represents the voltage or amplitude of the ECG waveforms or deflections. Voltage is measured in millivolts (mV). Voltage may appear as a positive or negative value because voltage is a force with direction as well as amplitude. Amplitude is measured in millimeters.

The default value for ECG machine calibration is 10 mm/mV. Thus when an ECG machine is calibrated correctly, a 1-mV electrical signal produces a deflection that measures precisely 10 mm tall (i.e., the height of 10 small boxes). When a calibration marker is present, it appears at the extreme left side of the ECG tracing, before the first waveform. Clinically, the height of a waveform is usually stated in millimeters rather than in millivolts. Proper calibration is critical when analyzing ST segments.

Consider This

Certain instances may warrant the use of a nonstandard calibration. For example, the calibration should be reduced if the ECG waveforms are too large to fit the page. Conversely, the calibration should be increased if the waveforms are too small to read. When changes in calibration are necessary, choose a calibration that will make interpretation easier; therefore, double the calibration if an increase in QRS size is needed. If a reduction in ECG size is necessary, halve the calibration. Always include a calibration pulse and note the change in calibration on the ECG printout.

A waveform (i.e., a deflection) is a movement away from the baseline in a positive (i.e., upward) or negative (i.e., downward) direction. Each waveform you see on an ECG is related to a specific electrical event in the heart. Waveforms are named alphabetically, beginning with P, QRS, T, and occasionally U. When electrical activity is not detected, a straight line is recorded. This line is called the **baseline** or **isoelectric line**. If the wave of depolarization (i.e., the electrical impulse) moves toward the positive electrode, the waveform recorded on ECG graph paper will be upright (i.e., a positive deflection). If the wave of depolarization moves away from the positive electrode, the waveform recorded will be inverted (i.e., a downward or negative deflection). A **biphasic** (i.e., partly positive, partly negative) waveform or a straight line is recorded when the wave of depolarization moves perpendicularly to the positive electrode. The term *equiphasic* may be used instead of *biphasic* to describe a waveform with no net positive or negative deflection.

A **complex** consists of several waveforms. A **segment** is a line between waveforms. It is named by the waveform that precedes or follows it. An **interval** is made up of a waveform and a segment. Normal waveforms, segments, and intervals are summarized in Tables 1.2 and 1.3.

TABLE 1.2	Waveforms and Complexes
ECG Component	**Physiology**
P wave	• Atrial depolarization • Normally 0.12 second (120 msec) or less • Normally no more than 2.5 mm in height
QRS complex	• Ventricular depolarization • Q wave is the first negative deflection, R wave is the first positive deflection, S wave is the first negative deflection after an R wave • Except for leads III and aVR, a normal Q wave in the limb leads is less than 0.03 second (30 msec) in duration. A pathologic Q wave is more than 0.03 second (30 msec) in duration or more than 30% of the height of the following R wave in that lead, or both (Anderson, 2020) • Normally 0.075 to 0.11 second (75 to 110 msec) in adults (Ganz & Link, 2020)
T wave	• Ventricular repolarization • Normally slightly asymmetric

ECG, Electrocardiogram.

TABLE 1.3	Segments and Intervals
ECG Component	**Physiology**
PR interval	• Conduction through atrial tissue, the AV junction, and the His-Purkinje system • Measures 0.12 to 0.20 second (120 to 200 msec) in adults; may be shorter in children and longer in older adults
ST segment	• Represents early ventricular repolarization • Normally isoelectric (i.e., flat) • Displacement (e.g., elevation, depression) is determined by identifying the onset of the QRS (the reference point) and then locating the J point, which is the point where the QRS complex and ST segment meet. Deviation is measured as the number of mm of vertical ST segment displacement (at the J point) from the reference point (Thygesen et al., 2018)
TP segment	• Represents the period of no electrical activity between the end of a PQRST cycle and the onset of the next • Normally isoelectric when the heart rate is within normal limits • Often unrecognizable with rapid heart rates
QT interval	• Reflects the onset of ventricular depolarization to the end of ventricular repolarization • Varies with age, sex, and heart rate • Generally, a normal QT interval is between 0.40 and 0.44 second

AV, Atrioventricular; *ECG,* electrocardiogram.

REFERENCES

Anderson, J. L., & Fang, J. C. (2020). ST elevation acute myocardial infarction and complications of myocardial infarction. In L. Goldman & A. I. Schafer (Eds.), *Goldman-Cecil medicine* (26th ed., pp. 388–401). Elsevier.

Ganz, L., & Link, M. S. (2020). Electrocardiography. In L. Goldman & A. I. Schafer (Eds.), *Goldman-Cecil medicine* (26th ed., pp. 246–253). Elsevier.

Shahoud, J. S., Ambalavanan, M., & Tivakaran, V. S. (2022). *Cardiac dominance.* StatPearls Publishing. https://www.ncbi.nlm.nih.gov/books/NBK537207/.

Thygesen, K., Alpert, J. S., Jaffe, A. S., Chaitman, B. R., Bax, J. J., Morrow, D. A., & White, H. D. (2018). Fourth universal definition of myocardial infarction. *Journal of the American College of Cardiology, 72*(18), 2231–2264.

QUICK REVIEW

Identify one or more choices that best complete the statement or answer the question.

1. In adults, a normal PR interval measures
   a. 0.04 to 0.10 second.
   b. 0.08 to 0.12 second.
   c. 0.12 to 0.20 second.
   d. 0.16 to 0.28 second.

2. The SA node and AV bundle are supplied by a branch of the _____ coronary artery in most individuals.
   a. right
   b. left main
   c. circumflex
   d. left anterior descending

3. Which of the following represents the period of no electrical activity between the end of a PQRST cycle and the onset of the next and is normally isoelectric when the heart rate is within normal limits?
   a. PR interval
   b. TP segment
   c. QT interval
   d. ST segment

4. The QRS complex
   a. normally follows each P wave.
   b. represents ventricular depolarization.
   c. normally measures 0.20 second or less.
   d. reflects conduction through atrial tissue and the AV junction.

5. Which of the following are used when analyzing ST-segment displacement on the ECG?
   a. Onset of the QRS complex and the J point
   b. Start of the P wave to the end of the T wave
   c. End of the T wave and the start of the next P wave
   d. Start of the P wave to the onset of the QRS complex

6. Which of the following correctly reflects examples of secondary pacemakers?
   a. SA node and AV junction
   b. SA node and Purkinje fibers
   c. AV junction and Purkinje fibers
   d. AV junction and left bundle branch

7. On the ECG, total ventricular activity is reflected by the
   a. TP segment.
   b. PR interval.
   c. QT interval.
   d. ST segment.

8. The myocardium is thickest in the
   a. left atrium.
   b. right atrium.
   c. left ventricle.
   d. right ventricle.

ANSWERS

1. **C.** In adults, the PR interval normally measures 0.12 to 0.20 second (120 to 200 msec). It may be shorter in children and longer in older adults.

2. **A.** The SA node receives its blood supply from the SA node artery that runs lengthwise through the center of the node. The SA node artery originates from the RCA in about 60% of people. The AV bundle is supplied by the RCA in 85% to 90% of the population. In the rest, the Cx provides the blood supply.

3. **B.** The TP segment represents the period of no electrical activity between the end of a PQRST cycle and the onset of the next and is normally isoelectric when the heart rate is within normal limits.

4. **A, B.** A QRS complex represents ventricular depolarization and normally follows each P wave. In adults, the normal duration of the QRS complex is 0.11 second or less.

5. **A.** ST-segment displacement (e.g., elevation, depression) is determined by identifying the onset of the QRS (the reference point) and then locating the J point, which is the point where the QRS complex and ST segment meet. The deviation is measured as the number of millimeters of vertical ST segment displacement (at the J point) from the reference point.

6. **C.** Secondary pacemaker sites include the cells of the AV junction and Purkinje fibers; their intrinsic rates are slower than that of the SA node.

7. **C.** The QT interval (which includes the QRS complex, ST segment, and T wave) represents total ventricular activity; this is the time from ventricular depolarization (i.e., activation) to repolarization (i.e., recovery).

8. **C.** The thickness of the myocardium varies from one heart chamber to another. This variation in thickness is related to the amount of resistance that must be overcome to pump blood out of the different chambers. For example, the atria encounter little resistance when pumping blood to the ventricles. As a result, the atria have a thin myocardial layer. On the other hand, the ventricles must pump blood to either the lungs (the right ventricle) or the rest of the body (the left ventricle). So, the ventricles have a much thicker myocardial layer than the atria. The wall of the left ventricle is thicker than that of the right because the left ventricle propels blood to most vessels of the body. The right ventricle moves blood only through the blood vessels of the lungs and then into the left atrium

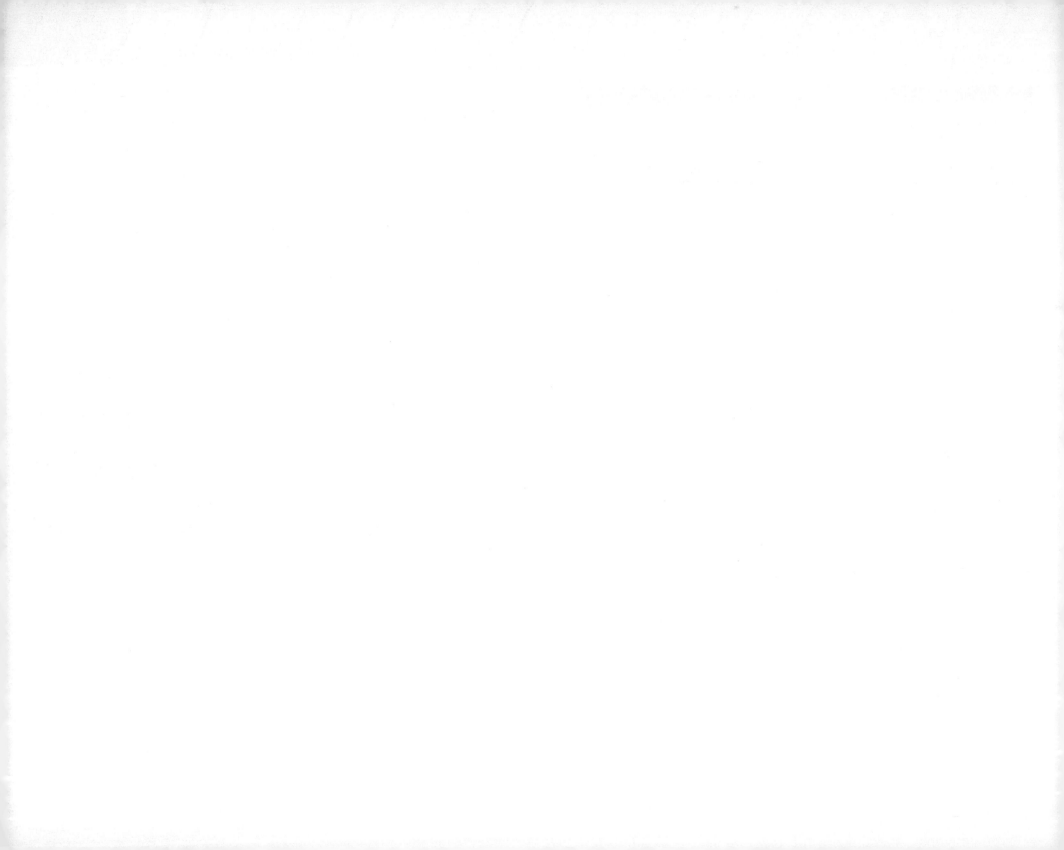

Leads, Axis, and Acquisition of the 12-Lead ECG

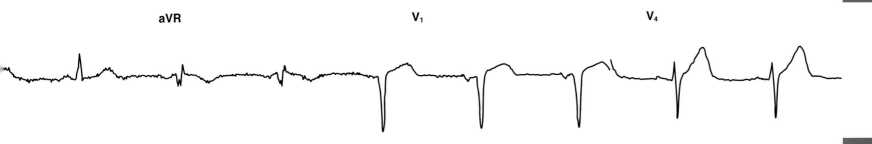

LEARNING OBJECTIVES

After reading this chapter, you should be able to:

1. Give examples of indications for using a 12-lead electrocardiogram (ECG).
2. Describe the correct anatomic placement of the standard limb leads, the augmented limb leads, and the chest leads.
3. Discuss the determination of the electrical axis using leads I and aVF.
4. Relate the cardiac surfaces or areas represented by the ECG leads.
5. Develop a reliable approach to quickly acquire a clear and accurate 12-lead ECG.
6. Explain the methods used to minimize the occurrence of artifact.
7. Recognize the importance of accurate lead placement before obtaining the ECG.
8. Understand the significance of frequency response in producing a reliable tracing.

KEY TERMS

artifact: Distortion of an ECG tracing by electrical activity that is noncardiac in origin

electrical axis: Net direction, or angle in degrees, in which the main vector of depolarization is pointed

electrode: An adhesive pad containing a conductive substance in the center that is applied to the patient's skin

frequency response: The spectrum in which an ECG can accurately reproduce the signals it is sensing

lead: A record (i.e., tracing) of electrical activity, specifically, the fluctuation in voltage differences between positive and negative electrodes

vector: Quantity having direction and magnitude, usually depicted by a straight arrow whose length represents magnitude and whose head represents direction

THE ELECTROCARDIOGRAM

An ECG detects and records current flow within the heart as measured on the body's surface. An **electrode** is an adhesive pad containing a conductive substance in the center that is applied to the patient's skin. The conductive media of the electrode conducts skin surface voltage changes through wires to a cardiac monitor. Electrodes are applied at specific locations on the patient's chest wall and extremities to view the heart's electrical activity from different angles and planes. One end of a monitoring cable, also called a *lead wire*, is attached to the electrode, and the other to an ECG machine. The cable conducts current back to the cardiac monitor.

A **lead** is a record (i.e., tracing) of electrical activity, specifically the fluctuation in voltage differences between positive and negative electrodes (Lederer, 2017). A standard 12-lead ECG uses 10 electrodes, 4 on the limbs and 6 on the chest wall, to record the heart's electrical activity from 12 angles. Each lead records the *average* current flow at a specific time in a portion of the heart. Box 2.1 lists examples of indications for obtaining a 12-lead ECG.

Frontal Plane Leads

Frontal plane leads view the heart from the front of the body as if it were flat. Six leads (leads I, II, III, aVR, aVL, and aVF) view the heart in the frontal plane (Fig. 2.1). Leads I, II, and III are called *bipolar* or *standard limb leads*. Leads aVR, aVL, and aVF are *unipolar* or *augmented limb leads*.

Consider This

A bipolar lead is an ECG lead that has a positive and negative electrode. Each lead records the difference between two selected electrodes' electrical potential (voltage). Leads I, II, and III are examples of bipolar leads. A unipolar lead consists of a single positive electrode and a reference point. The reference point (with zero electrical potential) lies in the center of the heart's electrical field (left of the interventricular septum and below the atrioventricular [AV] junction).

Box 2.1	Indications for Obtaining a 12-Lead Electrocardiogram
• Abdominal or epigastric pain • Assisting in dysrhythmia interpretation • Chest pain or discomfort • Diabetic ketoacidosis • Dizziness • Dyspnea • Electrical injuries • Known or suspected electrolyte imbalances	• Known or suspected medication overdoses • Right or left ventricular failure • Status before and after electrical therapy (e.g., defibrillation, cardioversion, pacing) • Stroke • Syncope or near syncope • Unstable patient, unknown etiology

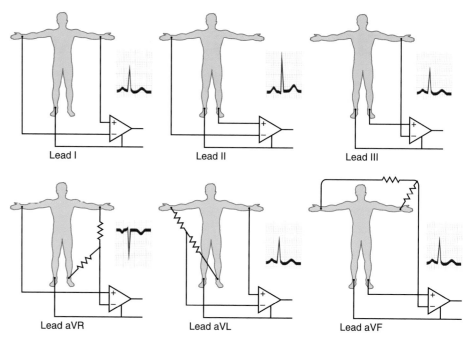

Fig. **2.1** Normal cardiac activation as shown in the limb leads. Under normal circumstances, P waves and QRS complex are typically upright in leads I, II, III, and aVF and inverted in aVR. In lead aVL, P waves are usually upright, although QRS complexes may be either upright or inverted. The right leg electrode serves to ground the system. (From Goldman, L., & Schafer, A. I. [2020]. *Goldman-Cecil medicine* [26th ed.]. Elsevier.)

Lead I compares the difference in electrical potential between the left arm (+) and right arm (−) electrodes. It views the lateral surface of the left ventricle. Lead II compares the difference in electrical potential between the left leg (+) and right arm (−) electrodes. It views the inferior surface of the left ventricle. Finally, lead III compares the difference in electrical potential between the left leg (+) and left arm (−) electrodes and views the left ventricle's inferior surface. Waveforms are usually positive in leads I, II, and III.

Leads aVR, aVL, and aVF are *augmented limb leads* that record measurements at a specific electrode with respect to a reference electrode. Frank Norman Wilson and colleagues used the term *central terminal* to describe a reference point that is the average of the limb lead electrical potentials. In the augmented leads, the Wilson central terminal (WCT) is calculated by the ECG machine's computer as an average potential of the electrical currents from the two electrodes other than the one being used as the positive electrode. For example, in lead aVL, the positive electrode is located on the patient's left arm. The ECG machine's computer calculates the central terminal by joining the electrical currents obtained from the electrodes on the patient's right arm and left leg. Lead aVL therefore represents the difference in electrical potential between the left arm and the central terminal. The electrical potential of the central terminal is essentially zero.

The electrical potential produced by the augmented leads is normally relatively small. The ECG machine augments (magnifies) the amplitude of the electrical potentials detected at each extremity by about 50% over those recorded at the standard limb leads. The "a" in aVR, aVL, and aVF refers to "augmented." The "V" refers to voltage, and the last letter refers to the position of the positive electrode. The "R" refers to the right arm, the "L" to the left arm, and the "F" to the left foot (i.e., leg).

Lead aVR views the endocardial surface of the ventricles from the right shoulder, which is the positive electrode. Because the wave of depolarization is moving away from lead aVR, waveforms in this lead are typically negative. Studies suggest that ST-segment elevation (STE) that is 1 mm or greater in lead aVR may be a significant indicator of left main coronary artery disease, proximal left anterior descending disease, or multivessel coronary artery disease (Sedighi et al., 2021; Thygesen et al., 2018; Uzun et al., 2020).

Lead aVL combines views from the right arm and the left leg, with the view being from the left arm and oriented to the lateral wall of the left ventricle. Waveforms observed in this lead are usually positive but may be biphasic (i.e., partly positive, partly negative). Lead aVF combines views from the right arm and the left arm toward the left leg; it views the inferior surface of the left ventricle from the left leg. Waveforms observed in this lead are usually positive but may be biphasic.

Horizontal Plane Leads

Six chest (precordial or "V") leads view the heart in the horizontal plane, allowing a view of the front and left side of the heart. The chest leads are unipolar and identified as V_1, V_2, V_3, V_4, V_5, and V_6. Each electrode in a "V" position is a positive electrode, measuring electrical potential with respect to the WCT (Fig. 2.2). The chest leads are summarized in Table 2.1.

When viewing the chest leads in a normal heart, the R wave becomes taller (i.e., increases in amplitude) and the S wave becomes smaller as the electrode is moved from right to left. This pattern is called *R-wave progression*. The *transition zone* is the area at which the amplitude of the R wave begins to exceed the amplitude of the S wave and usually occurs in the area of leads V_3 and V_4 (Ganz & Link, 2020).

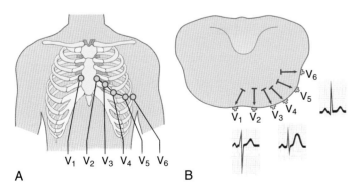

Fig. **2.2** Chest leads. (A) Positioning of the chest leads on the chest wall. (B) Normal cardiac activation as seen in the chest leads. (From Goldman, L., & Schafer, A. I. [2020]. *Goldman-Cecil medicine* [26th ed.]. Elsevier.)

TABLE **2.1**	Chest Leads	
Lead	Positive Electrode Position	Heart Area Viewed
V_1	Right side of sternum, fourth intercostal space	Interventricular septum
V_2	Left side of sternum, fourth intercostal space	Interventricular septum
V_3	Midway between V_2 and V_4	Anterior surface of left ventricle
V_4	Left midclavicular line, fifth intercostal space	Anterior surface of left ventricle
V_5	Left anterior axillary line, fifth intercostal space	Lateral surface of left ventricle
V_6	Left midaxillary line, fifth intercostal space	Lateral surface of left ventricle

Consider This

Electrode placement in the correct intercostal space is critical when evaluating R-wave progression.

LAYOUT OF THE 12-LEAD ECG

Look at the 12-lead ECG in Fig. 2.3. Notice that the standard limb leads are recorded in the first column, the augmented limb leads in the second column, and the chest leads in the third and fourth columns. The 12-lead ECG provides a 2.5-second view of each lead because it is assumed that 2.5 seconds is long enough to capture at least one representative complex. Although most 12-lead ECG machines acquire the signals for all leads at the same time, other machines obtain the signals sequentially (i.e., all limb leads, then the augmented limb leads, followed by leads V_1 through V_3, and finally leads V_4 through V_6). The 12-lead ECG machines used in the hospital setting typically record at least one rhythm strip at the bottom of the printout.

Note that the information printed on the upper left corner of Fig. 2.3 includes measurements of intervals in milliseconds (msec). This information is provided by the computer's interpretive program, which is usually very accurate when calculating heart rates, axes, and intervals.

Consider This

When a simultaneous tracing is obtained, the beats in a vertical column are all the product of the same ventricular depolarization. Likewise, beats in a horizontal row are continuous, even as the leads change.

Female   Caucasian

Room:
Loc:

Vent. rate	77 bpm
PR interval	156 msec
QRS duration	80 msec
QT/QTc	356/402 msec
P-R-T axes	73 56 60

Normal sinus rhythm
Normal ECG

Fig. **2.3**

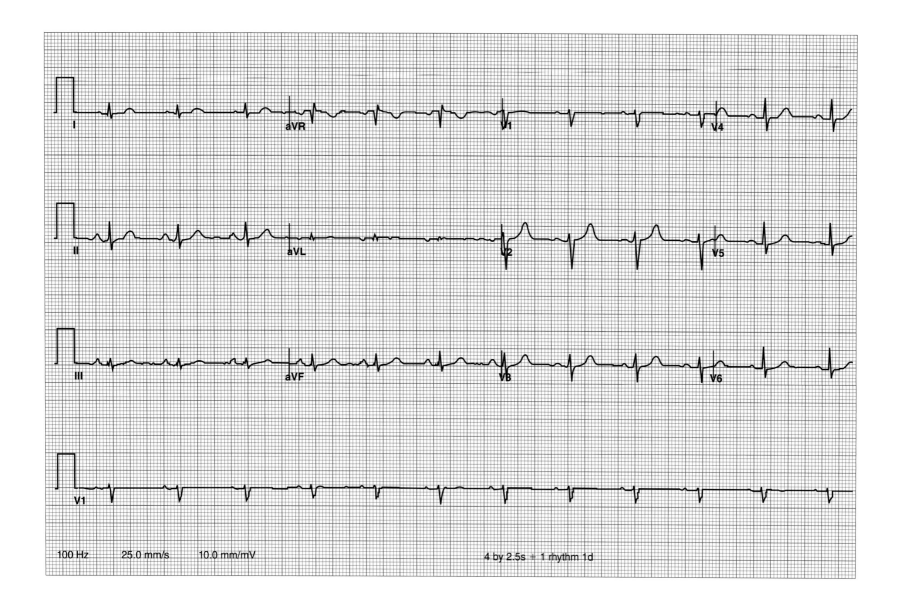

100 Hz   25.0 mm/s   10.0 mm/mV   4 by 2.5s + 1 rhythm 1d

Right Chest Leads

Other chest leads that are not part of a standard 12-lead ECG may be used to view specific heart surfaces. For example, right chest leads are used to evaluate the right ventricle when a right ventricular infarction is suspected (Fig. 2.4). Placement of right chest leads is identical to the placement of the standard chest leads, except it is done on the right side of the chest. If time does not permit obtaining all of the right chest leads, the lead of choice is V_4R. A summary of the right chest leads can be found in Table 2.2.

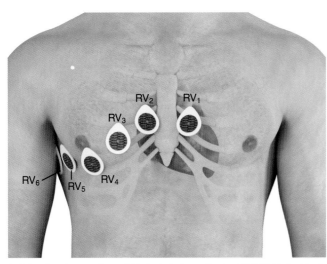

Fig. **2.4** Electrode locations for recording a right chest electrocardiogram (ECG). Right chest leads are not part of a standard 12-lead ECG but are used when a right ventricular infarction is suspected. (From Hedges, J. R., Custalow, C.B., & Thomsen, T. W. [2019]. *Roberts and Hedges' clinical procedures in emergency medicine and acute care* [7th ed.]. Elsevier.)

TABLE **2.2**	Right Chest Lead Placement
Lead	**Placement**
V_1R	Lead V_2
V_2R	Lead V_1
V_3R	Midway between V_2R and V_4R
V_4R	Right midclavicular line, fifth intercostal space
V_5R	Right anterior axillary line, fifth intercostal space
V_6R	Right midaxillary line, fifth intercostal space

Posterior Chest Leads

Posterior chest leads can be used to evaluate the heart's posterior surface when an infarction affecting this area is suspected. These leads are placed further left and toward the back. All the leads are placed on the same horizontal line as V_4 to V_6. Lead V_7 is placed at the posterior axillary line. Lead V_8 is placed at the angle of the scapula (i.e., the posterior scapular line) and lead V_9 is placed over the left border of the spine (Fig. 2.5).

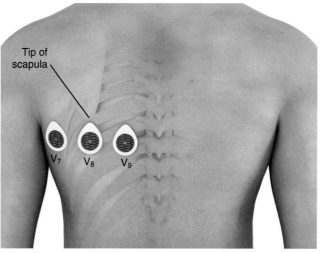

Fig. **2.5** Electrode locations for left posterior chest lead placement. (From Hedges, J. R., Custalow, C.B., & Thomsen, T. W. [2019]. *Roberts and Hedges' clinical procedures in emergency medicine and acute care* [7th ed.]. Elsevier.)

VECTORS AND AXIS

Leads have a negative (−) and positive (+) electrode pole that senses the magnitude and direction of the electrical force caused by the spread of waves of depolarization and repolarization throughout the myocardium. A **vector** (arrow) is a symbol representing this force. A vector's angle of orientation represents the average direction of current flow, and its length represents the voltage (i.e., amplitude). Leads that face the tip or point of a vector record a positive deflection on ECG paper.

An imaginary line joining the positive and negative electrodes of a lead is called the *axis* of the lead (Fig. 2.6). **Electrical axis** refers to the net direction, or angle in degrees, in which the primary depolarization vector is pointed. When *axis* is used by itself, it refers to the QRS axis.

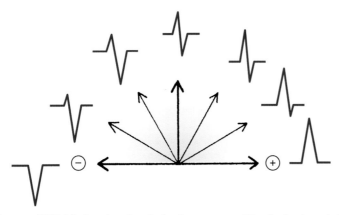

Fig. **2.6** The range of QRS deflections depends on the heart's average current flow direction *(arrows)* with respect to a lead's axis. The positive and negative circles represent the electrodes of a bipolar lead, and the straight, heavy line between them represents the lead's axis. The arrows represent seven possible current flow directions in the heart. (From Conover M. B. (1996). *Understanding electrocardiography* [7th ed.]. Mosby.)

During normal ventricular depolarization, the interventricular septum's left side is first stimulated. The electrical impulse then crosses the septum to stimulate the right side. The left and right ventricles are then depolarized simultaneously. Because the left ventricle is considerably larger than the right, right ventricular depolarization forces are overshadowed on the ECG.

The axes of leads I, II, and III form an equilateral triangle with the heart at the center (i.e., Einthoven's triangle). Einthoven's law states that the sum of the electrical currents recorded in leads I and III equals the sum of the electrical current recorded in lead II, which can be expressed as lead I + lead III = lead II. If the augmented limb leads are added to the equilateral triangle and the axes of the six leads moved in a way in which they bisect each other, the result is the *hexaxial reference system* (Fig. 2.7). The hexaxial reference system represents all of the frontal plane (limb) leads with the heart in the center and is the means used to express the location of the frontal plane axis. This system forms a 360-degree circle surrounding the heart. The positive end of lead I is designated at 0 degrees. The six frontal plane leads divide the circle into segments, each representing 30 degrees. All degrees in the upper hemisphere are labeled as negative degrees, and all degrees in the lower hemisphere are labeled as positive degrees.

In the hexaxial reference system, the axes of some leads are perpendicular. For example, lead I is perpendicular to lead aVF, lead II is perpendicular to lead aVL, and lead III is perpendicular to lead aVR. If the electrical force moves toward a positive electrode, a positive (upright) deflection will be recorded. If the electrical force moves away from a positive electrode, a negative (downward) deflection will be recorded. If the electrical force is parallel to a given lead, the largest deflection in that lead will be recorded. If the electrical force is perpendicular to a lead axis, the resulting ECG complex will be isoelectric and/or equiphasic in that lead. Notice that leads III and aVL are positioned on opposite (reciprocal) sides of the hexaxial reference system.

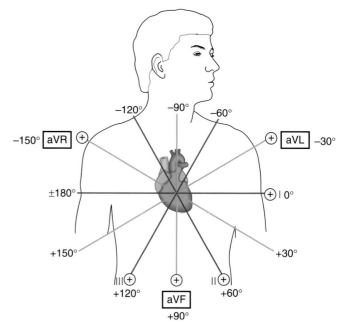

Fig. **2.7** The hexaxial reference system. (From Beachey, W. [2018]. *Respiratory care anatomy and physiology: Foundations for clinical practice* [4th ed.]. Elsevier.)

To determine the electrical axis, look again at Fig. 2.3. Because the hexaxial reference system is derived from the limb leads, we will focus on the leads shown in the two columns on the left side of the figure (leads I, II, III, aVR, aVL, and aVF). Look for the most equiphasic or isoelectric QRS complexes in these leads. Lead aVL shows QRS complexes that most closely reflect our criteria. The patient's QRS axis is perpendicular to the positive electrode in lead aVL. Look at the hexaxial reference system diagram (see Fig. 2.7) to determine which ECG lead is perpendicular to lead aVL. Lead II is perpendicular to lead aVL. Now we know that the patient's QRS axis is moving along the same vector as lead II. Note that the values associated with lead II in the hexaxial reference system diagram are –120 degrees and +60 degrees. To determine whether the QRS axis is moving in a positive or negative direction, look at lead II in Fig. 2.3 and determine whether the QRS complex is primarily positive or negative in this lead. You will see that the QRS is predominantly positive in lead II; therefore, this patient's QRS axis is about +60 degrees. At the top of Fig. 2.3, you will see the computer's calculation of the patient's P-QRS-T axes. The computer calculated the patient's QRS axis at +56 degrees. Our estimate of +60 degrees was very close!

In adults, the normal QRS axis is between –30 and +90 degrees in the frontal plane (Ganz & Link, 2020). Current flow to the right of normal is called *right axis deviation* (between +90 and ±180 degrees). Current flow in the direction opposite of normal is called *indeterminate*, "no man's land," *northwest*, or *extreme right axis deviation* (between

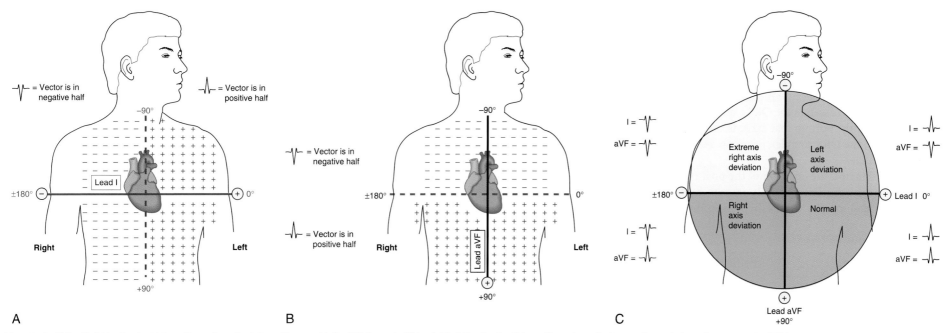

Fig. **2.8** (A) Lead I divides the chest into positive and negative halves with respect to the QRS it records. (B) Lead aVF divides the chest into positive and negative lower and upper halves with respect to the QRS it records. (C) Using leads I and aVF together locates the mean cardiac vector within a 90-degree quadrant. (From Beachey, W. [2018]. *Respiratory care anatomy and physiology: Foundations for clinical practice* [4th ed.]. Elsevier.)

−90 and ±180 degrees). Current flow to the left of normal is called *left axis deviation* (between −30 and −90 degrees).

Shortcuts exist to determine axis deviation. Leads I and aVF divide the heart into four quadrants (Fig. 2.8). These two leads can be used to quickly estimate the electrical axis. In leads I and aVF, the QRS complex is normally positive. If the QRS complex in either or both of these leads is negative, axis deviation is present (Table 2.3).

Right axis deviation may be a normal variant, particularly in children and young adults. Other causes of right axis deviation include mechanical shifts associated with inspiration or emphysema, right bundle branch block, right ventricular hypertrophy, chronic obstructive pulmonary disease (COPD), altered conduction pathways (e.g., Wolff-Parkinson-White [WPW] syndrome), lateral myocardial infarction (MI), left posterior fascicular block, ventricular dysrhythmias, and acute or chronic pulmonary thromboembolism. Extreme right axis deviation may be associated with emphysema, hyperkalemia, transposed ECG leads, ventricular dysrhythmias, or ventricular pacing.

Left axis deviation may be associated with age-related changes. Other causes of left axis deviation include mechanical shifts caused by an elevated diaphragm (e.g., obesity, pregnancy, ascites, abdominal tumors), altered conduction pathways (e.g., WPW syndrome), emphysema, hyperkalemia, prior inferior MI, left bundle branch block, left

TABLE **2.3**	Two-Lead Method of Axis Determination			
Axis	**Normal**	**Left**	**Right**	**Extreme Right**
Lead I QRS direction	Positive	Positive	Negative	Negative
Lead aVF QRS direction	Positive	Negative	Positive	Negative

anterior fascicular block, ventricular tachycardia, ventricular pacing, and left ventricular hypertrophy.

WHAT EACH LEAD "SEES"

Think of the positive electrode as an eye looking in at the heart. The part of the heart that each lead "sees" is determined by two factors. The first factor is the dominance of the left ventricle on the ECG, and the second is the position of the positive electrode on the body. Because the ECG does not directly measure the heart's electrical activity, it does not "see" all current flowing through the heart. What the ECG sees from its vantage point on the body's surface is the net result of countless individual currents competing in a tug-of-war. For example, the QRS complex, which represents ventricular depolarization, does not display all the electrical activity occurring in the right and left ventricles. Instead, it shows the net result of a tug-of-war produced by the many individual currents in both the right and left ventricles. Because the left ventricle is much larger than the right, the left overpowers it. What is seen in the QRS complex is the additional electrical activity of the left ventricle (i.e., the portion that exceeds the right ventricle). Therefore, in a normally conducted beat, the QRS complex primarily represents the electrical activity occurring in the left ventricle.

The second factor, the position of the positive electrode on the body, determines which portion of the left ventricle is seen by each lead. You can memorize the view of each lead, or you can easily reason it by remembering where the positive electrode is located. Fig. 2.9 demonstrates the portion of the left ventricle that each lead views.

Contiguous Leads

The sudden blockage of a coronary artery will result in myocardial ischemia, injury, and/or death of the area of the myocardium supplied by the affected artery. Remember that the positive electrode of each ECG lead is like an eye looking in at the heart. Therefore, every lead will not see and record the ECG changes associated with ischemia, injury, or infarction. If ECG findings are seen in leads that look directly at the area fed by the blocked vessel (i.e., facing leads), they are called *indicative changes* (Fig. 2.10). If ECG findings are seen in leads opposite the affected area, they are called *reciprocal changes*, discussed later.

Indicative changes are significant when they are seen in two *anatomically contiguous* leads. Two leads are contiguous if they look at the same or adjacent areas of the heart or if they are numerically consecutive chest leads. To better understand this, look at Table 2.4, which shows the area viewed by each lead of a standard 12-lead ECG. The colors in the table were added so that you can quickly see the areas of the heart viewed by the same leads. For example leads II, III, and aVF appear the same color in the table because they view the inferior wall of the left ventricle. Because these leads "see" the same part of the heart, they are considered contiguous leads.

Leads I, aVL, V_5, and V_6 are contiguous because they all look at adjoining tissue in the lateral wall of the left ventricle. Leads V_1 and V_2 are contiguous because both leads look at the septum. Leads V_3 and V_4 are contiguous because both leads look at the anterior wall of the left ventricle. Leads V_2 and V_3 are contiguous because they are numerically consecutive chest leads.

If right chest leads such as V_4R, V_5R, and V_6R are used, they are contiguous because they view the right ventricle. Leads V_7, V_8, and V_9 are contiguous because they look at the heart's posterior (i.e., inferobasal) surface.

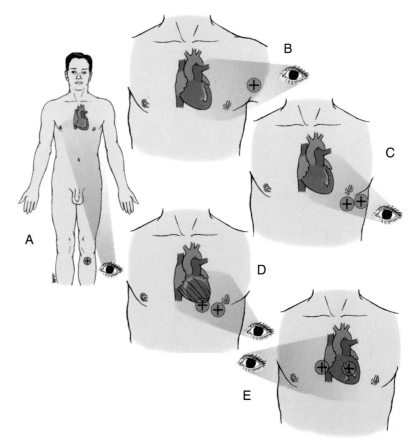

Fig. **2.9** Lead viewpoints. (A) Leads II, III, and aVF each have their positive electrode positioned on the left leg. From the perspective of the left leg, each "sees" the inferior wall of the left ventricle. (B) From their vantage point on the left arm, leads I and aVL "look" in at the lateral wall of the left ventricle. (C) Leads V_5 and V_6 also "view" the lateral wall because they are positioned on the axillary area of the left chest. (D) Leads V_3 and V_4 are positioned in the anterior chest area. From this perspective, these leads "see" the anterior wall of the left ventricle. (E) The septal wall is "seen" by leads V_1 and V_2, which are positioned next to the sternum. Lead aVR, which is not shown, views the heart from the right shoulder. It "sees" the basal ventricular septum and the inferior and lateral apex of the heart.

Reciprocal Leads

ECG changes associated with ischemia, injury, or infarction may be associated with reciprocal ("mirror image") ECG changes in leads opposite (i.e., about 180 degrees away from) the leads that show the indicative change (see Fig. 2.10). For example, STE in lead III, an indicative change, will show ST-segment depression, a reciprocal change, in lead aVL. Reasons why reciprocal changes may be subtle or may not be apparent on a standard 12-lead ECG include the following (Wagner et al., 2009):

- The standard 12-lead ECG may not reflect the leads opposite the indicative change.
- The magnitude of the voltage transmitted to the body surface is inadequate to meet diagnostic criteria. A low QRS voltage may be caused by conditions such as cardiomyopathy, diffuse coronary artery disease, COPD, hypothyroidism, and prior MI.
- The presence of confounding ECG abnormalities, such as intraventricular conduction disturbances.

Experts note that lead aVR does not have any contiguous leads; however, it is reciprocal to limb leads I and II and partly reciprocal to chest leads V_4, V_5, and V_6. For example, infarction of the upper portion of the interventricular septum can produce STE in aVR and ST depression in leads I, II, and V_4 through V_6.

Cabrera Display Format

The 12-lead ECG layout previously described has been used for many years worldwide. The national standard in Sweden is the Cabrera format, which has been used for more than 40 years. With this display format, the frontal plane leads are displayed in the logical sequence of impulse progression through the heart in the frontal plane and then in the horizontal plane (Fig. 2.11).

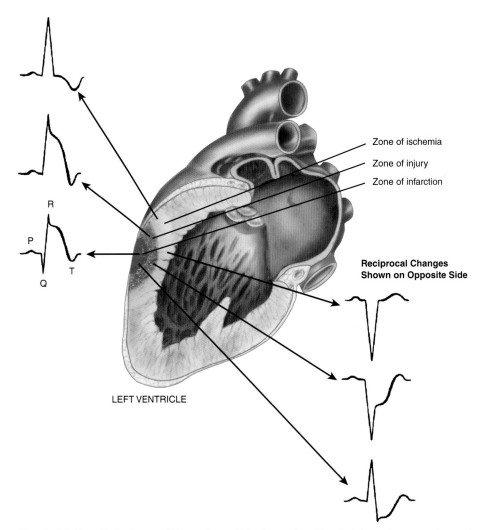

Zone of ischemia
Zone of injury
Zone of infarction

Reciprocal Changes Shown on Opposite Side

LEFT VENTRICLE

Fig. **2.10** Zone of ischemia, zone of injury, and zone of infarction are shown through electrocardiogram waveforms and reciprocal waveforms corresponding to each zone. (Modified from Urden, L. D., Stacy, K. M., & Lough, M. E. [2022]. *Critical care nursing: Diagnosis and management* [9th ed.]. Elsevier.)

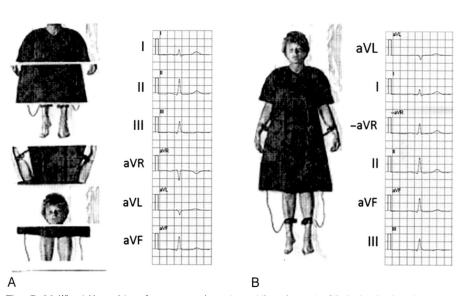

A   B

Fig. **2.11** When taking a picture of a person, one does not expect the various parts of the body to be shown in "jumbled" order (A) or even one of the subpictures shown upside down. This is akin to displaying the limb leads of the 12-lead ECG in the classical way. The Cabrera display (B) shows the limb leads in sequential, "anatomic" order. (From Lam, A., Wagner, G. S., & Pahlm, O. [2015]. The classical versus the Cabrera presentation system for resting electrocardiography: Impact on recognition and understanding of clinically important electrocardiographic changes. *Journal of Electrocardiology*, 48(4), 476–482).

TABLE **2.4**	Localizing Electrocardiogram Changes		
I: Lateral	aVR: —	V_1: Septum	V_4: Anterior
II: Inferior	aVL: Lateral	V_2: Septum	V_5: Lateral
III: Inferior	aVF: Inferior	V_3: Anterior	V_6: Lateral

Recall that a standard 12-lead ECG displays leads in the following sequence: I, II, III, aVR, aVL, aVF (frontal plane leads), V_1, V_2, V_3, V_4, V_5, and V_6 (horizontal plane leads). In contrast, the Cabrera format displays the frontal plane leads in anatomical sequence (i.e., aVL, I, −aVR, II, aVF, III), followed by the horizontal plane leads (i.e., V_1, V_2, V_3, V_4, V_5, and V_6). Note that the inverse form of lead aVR is used with the Cabrera format and is indicated as −aVR, which refers to lead aVR with reversed polarity. In the hexaxial reference system, the inverse form of lead aVR exists at 30 degrees in the frontal plane, filling the gap between lead I, which is at 0 degrees, and lead II, which is at 60 degrees.

Experts observe that potential advantages of the use of the Cabrera sequence include the following (Lam et al., 2015; Lindow et al., 2019):

- Identification of STE in two contiguous leads is simpler when contiguous leads are shown adjacent to each other.
- Viewing contiguous leads aids in understanding lead relationships and reciprocal changes.
- The inverted form of lead aVR can be viewed as a transition lead between the lateral (i.e., lead I) and inferior (i.e., lead II) areas of the heart, improving recognition of lateral and inferior ischemia and infarction and making the neglect of lead aVR unlikely.
- The electrical axis can be calculated faster and with greater accuracy.

The American Heart Association and the *American Journal of Cardiology* have recommended that all vendors of ECG machines provide the Cabrera system as an option (Wagner et al., 2009).

12-LEAD ECG ACQUISITION

The goals of 12-lead acquisition are to obtain an ECG that is free of distortion (clear), with the leads placed correctly (accurate), and done quickly (fast).

Goal 1: Clear

Accurate 12-lead ECG interpretation requires a tracing in which the waveforms and intervals are free of distortion. Distortion of an ECG tracing by electrical activity that is noncardiac in origin is called **artifact**, which may result from external or internal sources. The presence of artifact can interfere with a 12-lead machine's ability to acquire and/or interpret the ECG. Although artifact is sometimes easy to detect, it can mimic serious dysrhythmias (Fig. 2.12) resulting in incorrect interpretation and leading to unnecessary testing and treatment.

Studies show that interface between the patient's skin and the ECG electrode is a common artifact source. When preparing the patient's skin for electrode application, ensure that the areas where the electrodes will be applied are clean and dry. Because alcohol can dry the skin and reduce electrical flow, cleansing the intended electrode sites with soap and water is preferred; however, gauze or alcohol pads can be used

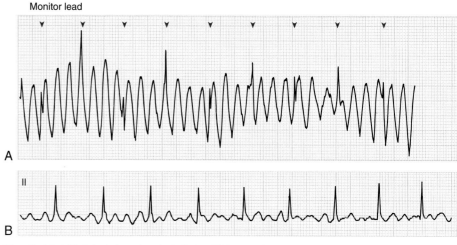

Fig. **2.12** Artifact simulating serious dysrhythmias. (A) Motion artifact mimicking ventricular tachyarrhythmia. Partly obscured normal QRS complexes *(arrowheads)* can be seen with a heart rate of approximately 100 beats/minute. (B) Parkinsonian tremor causing baseline oscillations mimicking atrial fibrillation. The regularity of QRS complexes may provide a clue to the source of this artifact. (From Libby, P., Bonow, R.O., Mann, D.L., Tomaselli, G.F., Bhatt, D.L., & Solomon, S.D. [2022]. *Braunwald's heart disease: A textbook of cardiovascular medicine* [12th ed.]. Elsevier.)

if the skin is oily or diaphoretic. Allow the skin to dry before applying electrodes. Lightly abrade the skin to remove dead skin cells, improve impulse transmission, and reduce motion artifact. Many electrode manufacturers include an abrasive area on the disposable backing of the electrode for this purpose, but skin prep tape or a gauze pad also work well.

When removing electrodes from their packaging, ensure that the conductive jelly in the center of the electrode is moist. If the electrode gel has dried out, it cannot penetrate the skin. As a result, the signal to the monitor will be weak, and artifact can result. Then, attach fresh electrodes to the lead wires *before* applying the electrodes to the skin. Doing so eliminates the patient discomfort caused by pressing the lead wires onto the electrode after placing them on the patient.

Internal artifact may result from patient movement, shivering, muscle tremors (e.g., seizures, Parkinson disease), hiccups, or medical devices such as a deep brain stimulator or left ventricular assist device.

A wandering baseline may occur because of patient movement. Subtle movements, such as those caused by the patient's breathing (particularly when electrodes have been applied directly over the ribs), talking, shivering, tapping toes, or rolling fingers, can be enough to produce artifact. Efforts to reduce muscle tension and the source of patient movement, such as having the patient relax and take a deep breath before ECG acquisition, can improve the tracing quality. When the tracing quality precludes a good interpretation, the tracing should be repeated.

Possible causes of external artifact include loose electrodes, broken ECG cables or lead wires, external chest compressions, and 60-cycle interference. Evaluation of the monitoring equipment (e.g., electrodes, cables, wires) before use and proper preparation of the patient's skin can minimize the problems associated with artifact. The signal from the patient's heart is conducted through lead wires and a cable to the monitor. If a lead wire is frayed or broken or the cable's insulation is cracked, the signal to the monitor is affected, and artifact can result. Inspect the monitoring cable and lead wires and replace them if damaged. If not preconnected, the limb lead and chest lead wires are inserted into a main cable, and the cable connector is inserted into the ECG port on the monitor.

Some electrical devices may interfere with the 12-lead monitor. If artifact persists after prepping the skin and troubleshooting did not turn up any problems, electromagnetic interference (EMI) might be the reason. The problem might be corrected by ensuring that power cords are not touching or lying near the ECG cable. EMI can also be affected by environmental factors such as nearby equipment, relative humidity, and static electricity.

Goal 2: Accurate

An accurate 12-lead ECG requires placing the electrodes correctly, positioning the patient, and selecting the correct settings for a diagnostic quality tracing. Although most 12-lead devices will default to the proper setting for these considerations, it is essential to understand the significance of each and be able to verify that they have been appropriately set.

Electrode Positioning

Although there are several indications for obtaining a 12-lead ECG, one of its most important uses is in triaging and diagnosing patients experiencing acute coronary syndromes (ACSs). Accurate positioning of electrodes is essential because ECG changes resulting from electrode misplacement can affect clinical decision-making and treatment.

The proper placement of limb electrodes has been debated for years, and there is considerable variability in clinical practice. It is common practice to use an alternative electrode configuration to reduce motion artifact from the extremities. With Mason-Likar electrode placement, the limb electrodes are moved to the torso, but chest electrode placement is unchanged. Although rhythm diagnosis is not adversely affected by Mason-Likar electrode placement, there is concern that Q waves in the inferior leads may be masked, making the detection of inferior infarction more difficult (Francis, 2016;

Sejersten et al., 2006). Another alternative electrode configuration is the Lund system, in which the limb electrodes are placed on the proximal areas of the limbs, and chest electrode placement is unchanged. An advantage of the Lund system is a reduction in movement-related artifact. In addition, the Lund system has been found to more closely replicate the ECG recordings obtained with conventional electrode positioning (Francis, 2016; Pahlm & Wagner, 2008).

Incorrect Electrode Positioning

Incorrect electrode placement is common. Examples of possible differences in interpretation with correct versus incorrect electrode placement are shown in Fig. 2.13. Most recording errors are the result of placing electrodes on the wrong extremity. However, transposing the lead wires in the monitoring cable can produce similar results (Greenfield, 2008). Reversal of the right and left arm lead wires is common (Fig. 2.14). Clues for detecting right arm/left arm electrode reversal include the following:

- Negative QRS complex in lead I
- Predominantly positive PQRST waveforms in lead aVR

Errors in the placement of the chest electrodes are common because their positioning is relative to anatomic landmarks. Obesity and the female anatomy are two variables that make consistent chest electrode positioning difficult (Harrigan et al., 2012). When placing chest electrodes on these patients, place the electrodes for leads V_3 through V_6 *under* the breast rather than *on* the breast.

The most common errors in chest electrode placement are positioning the V_1 and V_2 electrodes in the second or third rather than in the fourth intercostal space and placing the V_4 to V_6 electrodes too high on the lateral chest (Mirvis & Goldberger, 2022). In addition, placing the right chest electrodes too high on the chest can produce patterns that mimic those of anterior MI or an intraventricular conduction delay (Mirvis & Goldberger, 2022).

Patient Positioning

Ideally, a patient should be supine when the ECG is acquired. This position is preferred because it provides adequate support for the limbs so that muscle activity is minimal (Wung, 2017). However, if the patient is not supine when the tracing is obtained, note the patient's position on the 12-lead printout.

Body position changes (e.g., supine, side-lying, sitting upright, standing) can cause changes in the mean QRS, P wave, and T wave axes, as well as changes in waveform amplitude (e.g., P, QRS, and T waves) on the ECG recording. These shifts have been attributed to changes in the heart's anatomical orientation in the chest cavity, lung volume fluctuations, and shifts in the electrode contact with the skin. Research shows that ECG recordings obtained with patients in the supine and standing positions are comparable. In contrast, ECGs recorded in the reclining and sitting positions differ significantly from those recorded when supine and standing (Khare & Chawala, 2016).

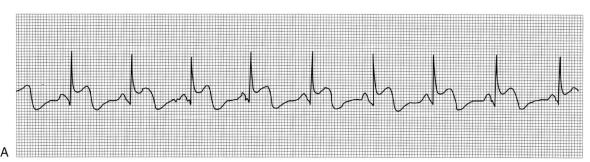

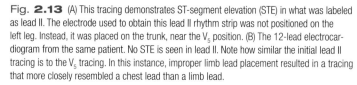

Fig. **2.13** (A) This tracing demonstrates ST-segment elevation (STE) in what was labeled as lead II. The electrode used to obtain this lead II rhythm strip was not positioned on the left leg. Instead, it was placed on the trunk, near the V_5 position. (B) The 12-lead electrocardiogram from the same patient. No STE is seen in lead II. Note how similar the initial lead II tracing is to the V_5 tracing. In this instance, improper limb lead placement resulted in a tracing that more closely resembled a chest lead than a limb lead.

A

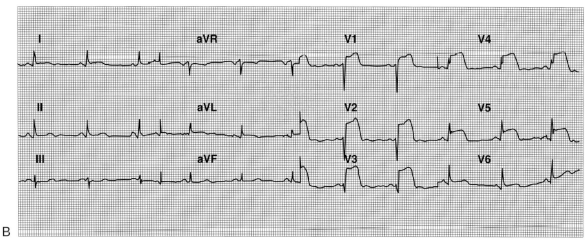

B

Frequency Response

The heart is not the only source of electrical activity that the ECG detects. Competing with the heart are such things as muscle tremors, movement artifact, 60-cycle interference, and other types of background "noise." Therefore, engineers work to produce a situation in which the monitor clearly sees the signal produced by the heart but ignores those signals that produce artifact.

To better understand this concept, once again, think of the ECG monitor as a voltmeter. Like any other voltmeter, it functions within a specific range or spectrum. If electrical activity occurs within that spectrum, the monitor senses it; if it occurs outside of the spectrum, the monitor does not sense it. The spectrum in which an ECG can accurately reproduce the signals it is sensing is referred to as the **frequency response**. Frequency response can be considered the window through which the ECG looks. If the window is wide, the ECG sees a lot; if the window is narrow, the ECG sees less. Fig. 2.15 demonstrates how changes in frequency response affect what the monitor can and cannot see.

Which is better? The answer depends on the purpose for which the ECG monitor is being used. A narrow frequency response can be referred to as *monitor quality*, and a wide frequency response can be referred to as *diagnostic quality*. Monitor quality aids in rhythm analysis, while diagnostic quality is necessary for accurate ST-segment analysis. The frequency response for *monitor* quality is often 0.05 Hertz (Hz, cycles per second) to 40 Hz. The frequency response for *diagnostic* quality is 0.05 to 150 Hz. The 12-lead machine's interpretive program uses ECG data obtained at this frequency when formulating its analysis.

Some slight variations among manufacturers and ECG models may be found. Newer monitors allow users to instantly switch between monitor quality and diagnostic quality. This feature enables health care professionals to use monitor quality when determining rate and rhythm and to switch to diagnostic quality for ST-segment analysis. The frequency response is printed on the ECG paper (see Fig. 2.3).

The ECG in Fig. 2.16 was obtained from a healthy 30-year-old emergency care provider. When recorded in monitor quality, the ST segment is elevated by about 2 mm in V_1.

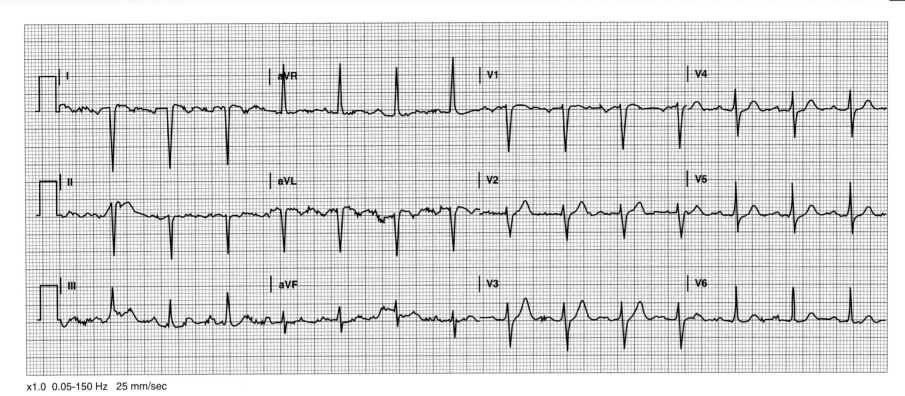

x1.0 0.05-150 Hz 25 mm/sec

Fig. **2.14** A 12-lead electrocardiogram showing reversed arm leads. Note the negative PQRST waveforms in lead I and the positive PQRST waveforms in lead aVR.

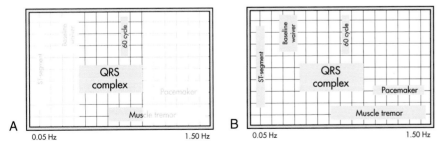

Fig. **2.15** (A) With a limited frequency response, the monitor can clearly "see" the QRS complex but cannot see the other features as clearly. (B) With a wider frequency response, the monitor can see the QRS complex and the ST segment as well.

While this tracing was being recorded, the monitor was switched from monitor quality to diagnostic quality. The fifth beat was the first to be captured in diagnostic quality. Notice that the ST segment is no longer elevated. ECG tracings obtained in monitor quality frequency response display STE that is not present in diagnostic quality, which could lead to misidentification of patients with ACS. Furthermore, the ST segment may appear normal in monitor quality but show STE when obtained in diagnostic quality. Also, note that there is more artifact in the later portion of the tracing. This example demonstrates the trade-off: increased fidelity often results in greater artifact.

Consider This

To use STE as an indicator of infarction, the monitor must be set to standard calibration and diagnostic quality.

Another example of how frequency response can change the ECG is demonstrated in Fig. 2.17. These strips were obtained within seconds of each other, first using monitor quality and then using diagnostic quality. A monitor-quality recording has produced STE beyond the amount present in a diagnostic quality tracing. In addition, the pacemaker spike is not obvious in the first tracing (monitor quality) but is prominent in the second tracing (diagnostic quality).

Fig. **2.16** The first four beats were obtained in monitor quality and demonstrate 2 mm of ST-segment elevation (STE). The fifth beat, obtained in diagnostic quality, shows no STE.

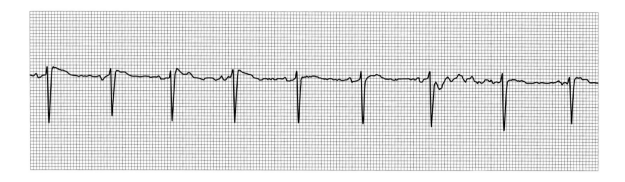

Fig. **2.17** (A) Tracing obtained in monitor quality. The patient's pacemaker was firing, but no pacemaker spikes were visible. The ST-segment elevation is prominent. (B) The same patient, with tracing obtained in diagnostic quality. The pacemaker spikes are now visible, as are some P waves with PR intervals that gradually lengthen.

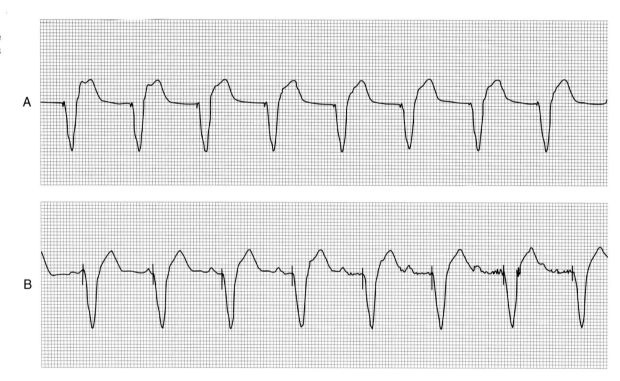

Goal 3: Fast

Because time is muscle when treating patients experiencing an ACS, much has to be accomplished in a short time. Fortunately, a 12-lead ECG can be obtained quickly. The speed of 12-lead ECG acquisition is particularly important to prehospital professionals because the goal is to be able to obtain a 12-lead ECG without an increase in scene time. The solution is to gain proficiency in the skill. As with virtually every other skill, 12-lead acquisition can be done more quickly with practice.

REFERENCES

Francis, J. (2016). ECG monitoring leads and special leads. *Indian Pacing Electrophysiology Journal, 16*(3), 92–95.

Ganz, L., & Link, M. S. (2020). Electrocardiography. In L. Goldman & A. I. Schafer (Eds.), *Goldman-Cecil medicine* (26th ed., pp. 246–253). Elsevier.

Greenfield, J. C., Jr. (2008). Erroneous electrocardiogram recordings because of switched electrode leads. *Journal of Electrocardiology, 41*(5), 376–377.

Harrigan, R. A., Chan, T. C., & Brady, W. J. (2012). Electrocardiographic electrode misplacement, misconnection, and artifact. *Journal of Emergency Medicine, 43*(6), 1038–1044.

Khare, S., & Chawala, A. (2016). Effect of change in body position on resting electrocardiogram in young healthy adults. *Nigerian Journal of Cardiology, 13*(2), 125–129.

Kligfield, P., Gettes, L. S., Bailey, J. J., Childers, R., Deal, B. J., Hancock, E. W., ..., Wagner, G. S. (2007). Recommendations for the standardization and interpretation of the electrocardiogram part I: The electrocardiogram and its technology. *Journal of the American College of Cardiology, 49*(10), 1109–1127.

Lam, A., Wagner, G. S., & Pahlm, O. (2015). The classical versus the Cabrera presentation system for resting electrocardiography: Impact on recognition and understanding of clinically important electrocardiographic changes. *Journal of Electrocardiology, 48*(4), 476–482.

Lederer, W. J. (2017). Cardiac electrophysiology and the electrocardiogram. In W. F. Boron & E. L. Boulpaep (Eds.), *Medical physiology* (3rd ed., pp. 483–506). Elsevier.

Lindow, T., Birnbaum, Y., Nikus, K., Maan, A., Ekelund, U., & Pahlm, O. (2019). Why complicate an important task?: An orderly display of the limb leads in the 12-lead electrocardiogram and its implications for recognition of acute coronary syndrome. *BMC Cardiovascular Disorders, 19*(1), 13.

Mirvis, D. M., & Goldberger, A. L. (2022). Electrocardiography. In P. Libby, R. O. Bonow, D. L. Mann, G. F. Tomaselli, D. L. Bhatt, & S. D. Solomon (Eds.), *Braunwald's heart disease: A textbook of cardiovascular medicine* (12th ed., pp. 141–174). Elsevier.

Omar, H. R., & Camporesi, E. M. (2014). The importance of lead aVR interpretation by emergency physicians. *American Journal of Emergency Medicine, 32*(10), 1289–1290.

Pahlm, O., & Wagner, G. S. (2008). Proximal placement of limb electrodes: A potential solution for acquiring standard electrocardiogram waveforms from monitoring electrode positions. *Journal of Electrocardiology, 41*(6), 454–457.

Sedighi, S., Fattahi, M., Dehghani, P., Aslani, A., Mehdipour Namdar, Z., & Hassanzadeh, M. (2021). aVR ST-segment changes and prognosis of ST-segment elevation myocardial infarction. *Health Science Reports, 4*(4), e387. doi:10.1002/hsr2.387.

Sejersten, M., Pahlm, O., Pettersson, J., Zhou, S., Maynard, C., Feldman, C. L., & Wagner, G. S. (2006). Comparison of EASI-derived 12-lead electrocardiograms versus paramedic-acquired 12-lead electrocardiograms using Mason-Likar limb lead configuration in patients with chest pain. *Journal of Electrocardiology, 39*(1), 13–31.

Thygesen, K., Alpert, J. S., Jaffe, A. S., Chaitman, B. R., Bax, J. J., Morrow, D. A., & White, H. D. (2018). Fourth universal definition of myocardial infarction. *Journal of the American College of Cardiology, 72*(18), 2231–2264.

Uzun, M., Kirilmaz, A., & Erinç, S. (2020). Lead aVR in electrocardiography: Clinical usefulness. *Hamidiye Medical Journal, 1*(1), 1–6. doi:10.4274/hamidiyemedj.galenos.2020.98608.

Vorobiof, G., & Ellestad, M. H. (2011). Lead aVR: Dead or simply forgotten? *JACC Cardiovascular Imaging, 4*(2), 187–190.

Wagner, G. S., Macfarlane, P., Wellens, H., Josephson, M., Gorgels, A., Mirvis, D. M., & Gettes, L. S. (2009). AHA/ACCF/HRS recommendations for the standardization and interpretation of the electrocardiogram: Part VI: Acute ischemia/infarction; a scientific statement from the American Heart Association Electrocardiography and Arrhythmias Committee. *Journal of the American College of Cardiology, 53*(11), 1003–1011.

Wung, S. F. (2017). Twelve-lead electrocardiogram. In D. J. Lynn-McHale Wiegand (Ed.), *AACN procedure manual for high acuity, progressive, and critical care* (7th ed., pp. 494–500). Elsevier.

QUICK REVIEW

Identify one or more choices that best complete the statement or answer the question.

1. Which of the following view the lateral surface of the left ventricle?
   a. Leads V_1 and V_2
   b. Leads V_3 and V_4
   c. Leads II, III, and aVF
   d. Leads I, aVL, V_5, and V_6

2. Which of the following are chest (i.e., precordial) leads?
   a. Leads I and aVL
   b. Leads I, II, and III
   c. Leads V_1, V_2, V_3, V_4, V_5, and V_6
   d. Leads I, II, III, aVR, aVL, and aVF

3. Where should the positive electrode for lead V_5 be positioned?
   a. Left midaxillary line at same level as V_4
   b. Left anterior axillary line at same level as V_4
   c. Left side of sternum, fourth intercostal space
   d. Right side of sternum, fourth intercostal space

4. Which of the following are clues for detecting right arm/left arm electrode reversal?
   a. A negative QRS complex in lead I
   b. A negative QRS complex in lead aVF
   c. Negative P waves in leads I, II, and III
   d. Predominantly negative PQRST waveforms in lead III
   e. Predominantly positive PQRST waveforms in lead aVR

5. In the hexaxial reference system, lead I is perpendicular to lead
   a. II.
   b. III.
   c. aVF.
   d. aVL.

6. Which leads look at adjoining tissue in the anterior region of the left ventricle?
   a. V_2, V_3, V_4
   b. II, III, aVF
   c. I, aVL, V_5
   d. aVR, aVL, aVF

7. When leads I and aVF are used to determine electrical axis, left axis deviation is present if the QRS is
   a. positive in lead I and positive in lead aVF.
   b. positive in lead I and negative in lead aVF.
   c. negative in lead I and negative in lead aVF.
   d. negative in lead I and positive in lead aVF.

8. Which of the following are bipolar leads?
   a. Leads I and aVL
   b. Leads I, II, and III
   c. Leads V_1, V_2, V_3, V_4, V_5, and V_6
   d. Leads I, II, III, aVR, aVL, and aVF

ANSWERS

1. **D.** Leads I, aVL, V_5, and V_6 view the lateral surface of the left ventricle.

2. **C.** Six chest (i.e., precordial or "V") leads view the heart in the horizontal plane. The chest leads are identified as V_1, V_2, V_3, V_4, V_5, and V_6.

3. **B.** Lead V_4 is recorded with the positive electrode in the left midclavicular line in the fifth intercostal space. Lead V_5 is recorded with the positive electrode in the left anterior axillary line at the same level as V_4.

4. **A, E.** Clues for detecting right arm/ left arm electrode reversal include (1) a negative QRS complex in lead I and (2) predominantly positive PQRST waveforms in lead aVR.

5. **C.** In the hexaxial reference system, the axes of some leads are perpendicular to each other. Lead I is perpendicular to lead aVF. Lead II is perpendicular to aVL, and lead III is perpendicular to lead aVR.

6. **A.** Leads V_2, V_3, and V_4 are next to each other on the patient's chest. Leads V_1 and V_2 view the septum. Leads V_3 and V_4 look at the anterior wall of the left ventricle. Therefore, leads V_2, V_3, and V_4 look at adjoining tissue in the anterior region of the left ventricle.

7. **B.** Leads I and aVF divide the heart into four quadrants. These two leads can be used to quickly estimate the electrical axis. If the QRS is positive in lead I and negative in lead aVF, left axis deviation is present.

8. **B.** Leads I, II, and III are bipolar leads. The augmented leads (aVR, aVL, and aVF) and chest leads (V_1, V_2, V_3, V_4, V_5, and V_6) are unipolar.

Acute Coronary Syndromes

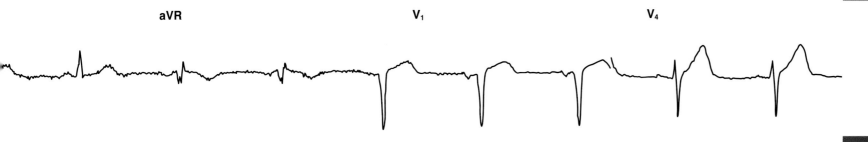

aVR   V₁   V₄

LEARNING OBJECTIVES

After reading this chapter, you should be able to:

1. Describe the pathophysiology of ischemic heart disease (IHD).
2. Differentiate the characteristics of stable (classic) angina, unstable angina (UA), and acute myocardial infarction (MI).
3. Recognize the electrocardiographic (ECG) changes produced by myocardial ischemia, injury, and infarction.
4. Localize the area of MI and predict which coronary artery is occluded.
5. Explain the importance of the 12-lead ECG in acute coronary syndromes (ACSs).
6. Discuss the three groups used when categorizing the ECG findings of the patient experiencing an ACS.

KEY TERMS

anginal equivalents: Symptoms of myocardial ischemia other than chest pain or discomfort

transmural MI: An MI extending from the endocardium to the epicardium

ISCHEMIC HEART DISEASE

Atherosclerosis is a systemic disease that results from a gradual buildup of deposits (plaque) in an artery's innermost (i.e., endothelial) layer. Large- and middle-sized arteries such as the aorta; coronary arteries; carotid and vertebral arteries; and the renal, iliac, and femoral arteries are often the most heavily affected.

An atherosclerotic plaque consists of lipids (mainly cholesterol), calcium, fibrin, and cellular waste products. These plaques differ regarding their vulnerability to rupture and their tendency to form a blood clot. As the plaque enlarges, it protrudes into the arterial lumen, partially or completely obstructing blood flow through the affected vessel. An atheromatous plaque blocking or gradually narrowing one or more epicardial coronary arteries is the most common cause of IHD.

Narrowing or blockage of a coronary artery can disrupt the oxygen supply to the area of the heart supplied by the affected vessel(s). Clinical symptoms can vary depending on the extent of occlusion and the speed at which it develops (Fig. 3.1) (Damjanov, 2017). Additional factors, such as endothelial dysfunction, microvascular disease, and vasospasm, may exist alone or in combination with coronary atherosclerosis and may be the primary cause of myocardial ischemia in some patients (Morrow & de Lemos, 2022) (Fig. 3.2).

An ACS is usually caused by atherosclerotic plaque rupture or erosion and thrombus formation leading to reduced coronary artery blood flow and distal myocardial ischemia (Atwood, 2022). If the cause of the ischemia is not reversed and blood flow is not restored to the affected area of the heart muscle, ischemia may lead to cellular injury and, ultimately, cellular death (i.e., infarction). Clinical presentations of IHD may include angina pectoris, silent myocardial ischemia, acute MI, or sudden cardiac death. Early assessment and emergency care are essential to prevent worsening ischemia.

Angina pectoris is chest discomfort caused by myocardial ischemia. It typically occurs because of an imbalance between myocardial oxygen demand (i.e., increased myocardial oxygen requirements) and myocardial oxygen supply (i.e., decreased coronary blood flow). Angina most often occurs in patients with coronary artery disease (CAD) involving at least one coronary artery, but it can be present in patients with normal coronary

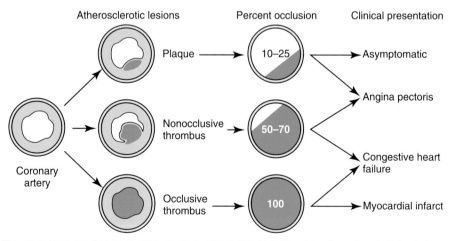

Fig. **3.1** Narrowing of a coronary artery may cause different clinical symptoms depending on the extent of occlusion and the speed at which it develops. (From Damjanov, I., Perry, A.M., & Perry, K.D. [2022]. *Pathology for the health professions* [6th ed.]. Elsevier.)

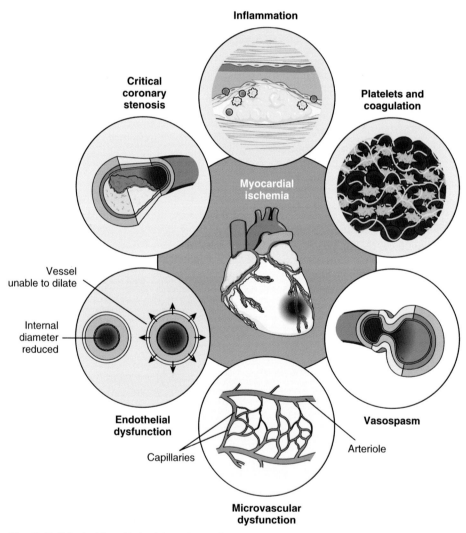

Fig. **3.2** Pathophysiology of ischemic heart disease. (From Libby, P., Bonow, R.O., Mann, D. L., Tomaselli, G.F., Bhatt, D.L., & Solomon, S.D. [2022]. *Braunwald's heart disease: A textbook of cardiovascular medicine* [12th ed.]. Elsevier.)

arteries. Angina also occurs in persons with uncontrolled hypertension, hypertrophic cardiomyopathy, or valvular heart disease.

Clinical Features

Although ischemic chest discomfort can occur anywhere in the chest, neck, arms, or back, it usually begins in the central or left chest and then radiates to the arm (especially the little finger [ulnar] side of the left arm), the wrist, the jaw, the epigastrium, the left shoulder, or between the shoulder blades. Anginal symptoms gradually intensify over a few minutes (Gulati et al., 2021). Common words used by patients experiencing angina to describe the sensation they are feeling are shown in Box 3.1.

Consider This

Not all chest discomfort is cardiac related. Therefore, obtaining an accurate history is essential to help determine if a patient's signs and symptoms are most likely related to ischemia secondary to CAD.

Although chest discomfort is the classic symptom associated with IHD, **anginal equivalents** (i.e., symptoms of myocardial ischemia other than chest pain or discomfort) may be present. Box 3.2 lists examples of anginal equivalents.

Anginal equivalents are common, particularly in older adults, individuals with diabetes, and people assigned female at birth. Although most older adults experience chest heaviness,

Box 3.1	Words Patients Often Use to Describe Angina

"Burning"
"Bursting"
"Constricting"
"Crushing"
"Grip-like"
"Heaviness"
"Indigestion-like"
"Pressing"
"Pressure-like"
"Squeezing"
"Strangling"
"Suffocating"
"Tightness"
"Uncomfortable numbness"
"A band across my chest"
"A vise tightening around my chest"
"A weight in the center of my chest"

Box 3.2	Examples of Anginal Equivalents

- Abdominal or epigastric discomfort
- Acute change in mental status
- Difficulty breathing
- Dizziness
- Dysrhythmias
- Excessive sweating
- Generalized weakness
- Isolated arm or jaw pain
- Lightheadedness
- Palpitations
- Shoulder or back pain
- Sudden fatigue
- Syncope or near-syncope
- Unexplained nausea or vomiting

pressure, or a squeezing sensation, more than 20% present without chest pain (Magidson, 2022). Consider the possibility of an ACS when an older adult experiences symptoms such as shortness of breath, syncope, weakness, a change in mental status, unexplained nausea, abdominal or epigastric discomfort, or an unexplained fall. In addition, older adults are more likely to present with more severe preexisting conditions, such as hypertension, heart failure, or a previous acute MI, than younger patients.

Individuals with diabetes may present atypically because of autonomic neuropathy, which affects the sensory innervation of the heart. Common signs and symptoms include generalized weakness, syncope, lightheadedness, or a change in mental status.

People assigned female at birth who experience an ACS are more likely than those assigned male at birth to present without chest pain (Brown, 2022). Among women presenting without chest pain, anginal equivalent symptoms commonly reported include pain in the upper back, neck, or jaw; difficulty breathing; weakness; and unusual fatigue. Interestingly, the pathophysiology of ACS may also differ by sex. For example, whereas plaque erosion is the most common cause of ACS in women, the cause is usually plaque rupture in men (Costello & Younis, 2020).

Consider This

Spontaneous coronary artery dissection, an uncommon cause of ACS, is a condition where a tear occurs in an epicardial coronary artery. Most (90%) cases involve people assigned female at birth (Brown, 2022), with few or no heart disease risk factors. Although its exact cause is unknown, predisposing factors that increase coronary artery well stress include inherited connective tissue diseases, systemic inflammatory conditions, pregnancy, multiparity, emotional stress, and fibromuscular dysplasia, a condition that causes abnormal cell growth in the arterial walls, leading to vessel narrowing, blockages, or tearing.

Diagnosis

Possible diagnostic studies that may be obtained in a patient with a complaint of chest discomfort include laboratory tests (including cardiac biomarkers), a 12-lead ECG, a chest radiograph, and echocardiography. In addition, noninvasive stress testing or coronary angiography, or both, may be performed to identify the amount of ischemic myocardium and establish a treatment plan.

The 12-lead ECG is an essential diagnostic tool for patients presenting with ischemic chest discomfort or anginal equivalent symptoms. The first 12-lead ECG should be obtained and interpreted within 10 minutes of patient contact. Obtain a repeat 12-lead ECG when clinically indicated by a change in patient condition.

Because ischemia affects repolarization, its effects can be viewed on the ECG as changes in ST segments and T waves (Fig. 3.3). When measured at the J point, an ST-segment depression of 0.5 mm or more is suggestive of myocardial ischemia when viewed in two or more anatomically contiguous leads (Thygesen et al., 2018). In addition, negative (i.e., inverted) T waves may also be present. After the episode of chest discomfort is resolved, ST segments usually return to the baseline.

Stable Angina

Stable (i.e., classic) angina remains relatively constant and predictable in terms of severity, signs and symptoms, precipitating events, and response to treatment. It is characterized by brief episodes of chest discomfort related to activities that increase the heart's need for oxygen. Common precipitating events and possible related signs and symptoms are shown in Box 3.3. Symptoms typically last less than 5 minutes and are usually relieved with rest (decreasing myocardial oxygen demand), short-acting nitroglycerin (NTG) (improving myocardial oxygen supply), or both.

Vasospastic Angina

Vasospastic angina (VA), also called *Prinzmetal angina* or *Prinzmetal variant angina*, is a form of angina caused by spasms of one or more epicardial coronary arteries. Patients with VA are generally younger and have fewer coronary risk factors (except for smoking) than patients with stable angina.

VA usually occurs at rest, often at night or in the early morning. Episodes may occur in clusters of two or three within 30 to 60 minutes. Although symptoms typically last only a few minutes, they are often described as severe. They may be accompanied by nausea, sweating, and syncope. Prolonged spasms may lead to subendocardial or **transmural MI** (i.e., extending from the endocardium to the epicardium), atrioventricular (AV) block, supraventricular or ventricular dysrhythmias, and, possibly, sudden cardiac death.

Smoking is an important predisposing risk factor for VA. In addition, there are reports of a possible association of VA with migraine headaches and Raynaud phenomenon, suggesting a possible association with a more generalized vasospastic disorder. Potential triggers to the onset of coronary spasm include emotional stress, cigarette smoking, use of central nervous system stimulants (e.g., cocaine), alcohol consumption, cold exposure, hyperventilation, magnesium deficiency, and medications (e.g., antimigraine agents, chemotherapy, anesthetics, antibiotics).

Recall that ECG changes observed with classic angina include ST-segment *depression*. However, VA usually produces ST-segment *elevation* (STE) during anginal episodes. Chest discomfort and ECG changes may resolve spontaneously or can be relieved by NTG. After the episode is resolved, ST segments usually return to the baseline. Because NTG effectively relieves coronary spasm, the ECG evidence of VA may be lost if no pretreatment ECG is obtained.

A multilead ECG showing STE in leads supplied by the left coronary artery (LCA) is shown in Fig. 3.4. This tracing was obtained a few moments before the administration of NTG. The patient reported that the NTG relieved the chest pain, and a second tracing was obtained. The obvious STE noted in the first example is no longer present, suggesting the possibility of VA (Fig. 3.5).

Experts caution that relief of symptoms with NTG administration should not be considered a diagnostic criterion for myocardial ischemia because other conditions (e.g., esophageal spasm) can demonstrate a similar response (Gulati et al., 2021). Therefore, considering the patient's clinical picture, history, cardiovascular risk factors, and so on, cannot be overemphasized when managing these patients.

Microvascular Angina

Angina sometimes occurs in the absence of significant atherosclerosis or vasospasm of the epicardial coronary arteries. With microvascular angina, angina is related to disease of the small, distal branches of the coronary arteries (i.e., coronary microvascular disease). Ischemia and angina occur because functional and structural changes in the coronary microvasculature disrupt the ability of the vessels to dilate and increase coronary blood flow in response to increased myocardial oxygen demand (Chen et al., 2016). Possible contributing factors of this type of angina include increased systemic inflammation, insulin resistance, abnormal vasoconstriction and impaired vasodilation of the microvascular bed, estrogen deficiency, and increased cardiac pain sensitivity, among others. Those at increased risk for microvascular dysfunction are women, individuals with hypertension, and individuals with diabetes and other insulin-resistant conditions (Gulati et al., 2021). Antiischemic therapy with beta-blockers and angiotensin-converting enzyme inhibitors, in addition to statins and lifestyle changes, have improved the quality of life in some patients (Gulati et al., 2021).

ACUTE CORONARY SYNDROMES

ACSs include UA, ST-elevation MI (STEMI), and non-ST-elevation MI (NSTEMI). If a coronary artery obstruction is partial or intermittent, the patient may experience no signs and symptoms (i.e., silent ischemia), UA, NSTEMI, or, possibly, sudden death. UA and NSTEMI differ primarily by whether myocardial ischemia is severe enough to cause cellular damage leading to detectable quantities of cardiac biomarkers (Amsterdam et al., 2014). Complete blockage of a coronary artery may result in STEMI or sudden

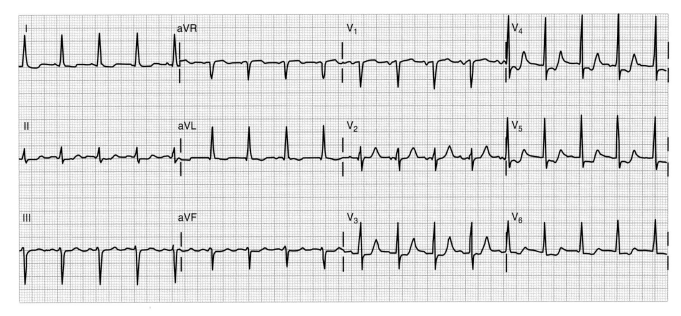

Fig. **3.3** Electrocardiogram obtained (A) during angina and (B) after administering sublingual nitroglycerin and subsequent resolution of angina. During angina, transient ST-segment depression and T-wave abnormalities are present. (From Benjamin, I. J., Griggs, R. C., Wing, E. J., & Fitz, J. G. [2016]. *Andreoli and Carpenter's Cecil essentials of medicine* [9th ed.]. Saunders.)

A

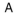

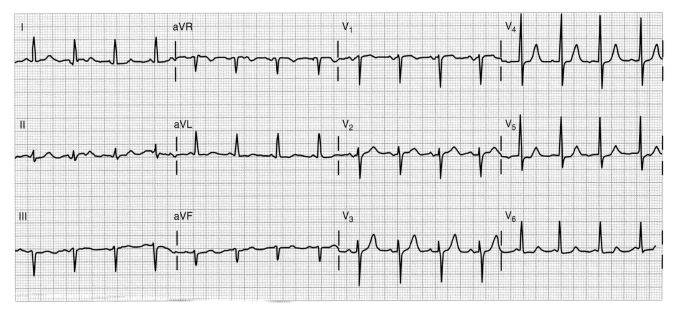

B

Box 3.3	Stable Angina Pectoris

COMMON PRECIPITATING EVENTS
- Emotional upset
- Exercise/exertion
- Exposure to cold weather
- Ingestion of a heavy meal

RELATED SIGNS AND SYMPTOMS
- Shortness of breath
- Palpitations
- Sweating
- Nausea or vomiting

death. Although NSTEMI and STEMI are life-threatening, they are discussed separately because their management strategies differ.

Consider This

Cardiac biomarkers are elevated when an infarction is present; they are not elevated in patients with UA because there is no tissue death.

The subendocardial area is the innermost half of the myocardium, and the subepicardial area is the outermost half (Fig. 3.6). The endocardial and subendocardial areas of the myocardial wall are the least perfused areas of the heart and the most vulnerable to ischemia because these areas have a high oxygen demand and are fed by the most distal branches of the coronary arteries. Recall that *transmural* is a term used to describe ischemia, injury, or infarction that extends from the endocardium to the epicardium. Therefore, a transmural MI describes an infarction involving the entire thickness of the left ventricular wall.

When a coronary artery is blocked, the region of the heart supplied by the affected artery is called the *area at risk* (Fig. 3.7). Ischemia occurs immediately in the area supplied by the affected artery. Anaerobic metabolism ensues, and lactic acid accumulates in the cardiac cells, quickly resulting in a loss of myocardial contractility. Ischemia also contributes to dysrhythmias, probably by causing electrical instability of ischemic areas of the heart (Mitchell & Connolly, 2021).

If blood flow is not restored to the affected artery, myocardial cells within the subendocardial area begin to reveal signs of injury within 20 to 40 minutes. However, if blood flow is quickly restored, the area at risk can potentially be salvaged; aerobic metabolism can resume, cellular repair can begin, and myocardial contractility can be restored.

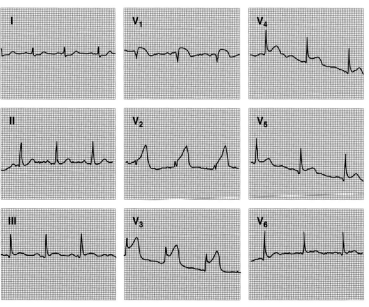

Fig. **3.4** A multilead electrocardiogram showing ST-elevation in leads supplied by the left coronary artery. This tracing was obtained a few moments before administering nitroglycerin.

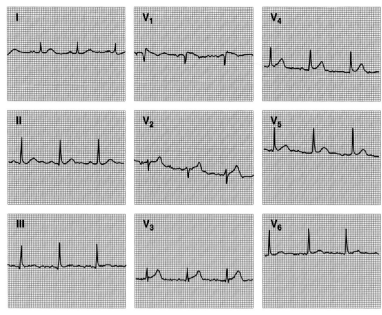

Fig. **3.5** Electrocardiogram obtained after nitroglycerin administration.

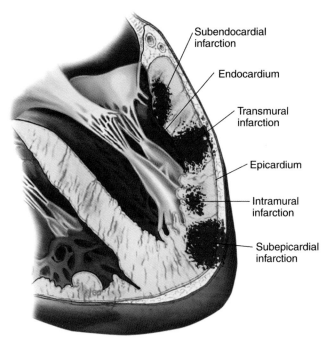

Fig. **3.6** Possible locations of infarctions in the ventricular wall. (From Urden, L. D., Stacy, K. M., & Lough, M. E. [2022]. *Critical care nursing: Diagnosis and management* [9th ed.]. Elsevier.)

Death of myocardial cells occurs when the area at risk has been deprived of blood flow for an extended interval, usually 2 to 4 hours or longer, depending on factors such as the presence of collateral circulation to the ischemic area, persistent or intermittent coronary vessel blockage, the metabolic/oxygen needs of the myocardium at risk, and the sensitivity of the myocardial cells to ischemia (Mitchell & Connolly, 2021; Thygesen et al., 2018).

Without clinical intervention (i.e., reperfusion therapy), the infarction can expand to involve the entire thickness of the myocardial wall; therefore, time is muscle when caring for patients with an ACS. The benefits of reperfusion therapy are greatest when performed early.

Diagnosis

The diagnosis of an ACS is made based on the following: (1) the patient's history and clinical presentation, (2) cardiac biomarker results, and (3) the patient's ECG findings (Fig. 3.8).

Clinical Features

The patient's clinical presentation and outcome depend on factors that include the following:
- Amount of myocardium supplied by the affected artery
- Severity and duration of myocardial ischemia
- Electrical instability of the ischemic myocardium
- Rate of development, degree, and duration of coronary obstruction
- Presence (and extent) or absence of collateral coronary circulation

The patient experiencing an ACS typically complains of retrosternal pain, pressure, heaviness, or tightness lasting 10 minutes or longer, usually occurring at rest or with minimal exertion.

Obtain a focused history, asking targeted questions to determine the patient's probability of an ACS. For example, ascertain the patient's presenting symptoms, including onset (abrupt or gradual) and duration, precipitating and relieving factors, location and radiation, cardiovascular risk factors, and associated symptoms. Additional complaints may include weakness, lightheadedness, palpitations, nausea, vomiting, sleep disturbances, or syncope. Exertional dyspnea is a common anginal equivalent in older adults. If the patient has a history of IHD, ask them to compare this episode with previous events.

Perform a physical examination. The patient experiencing an ACS may appear anxious, pale, or diaphoretic. Whereas patients with angina often remain still because activity increases their chest discomfort, some patients experiencing STEMI appear restless and move about to relieve their symptoms (Scirica et al., 2022). The heart rate can vary from within the expected range to slow or rapid. The blood pressure is typically normal but may be elevated because of pain and anxiety. Heart sounds, particularly S_1, may be muffled. An S_4 is common, and an S_3 may be heard in individuals with heart failure. During the physical examination, consider the possibility of other conditions that can cause chest pain or discomfort, such as acute pericarditis, aortic dissection, cardiac tamponade, gastroesophageal reflux, pneumonia, pneumothorax, and pulmonary embolism.

Cardiac Biomarkers

Cardiac biomarkers help confirm the diagnosis of MI for patients with STEMI. They are also helpful in confirming the diagnosis of MI when patients present without STE on their ECG, when the diagnosis may be unclear, and in distinguishing patients with UA from those with NSTEMI.

Cardiac troponins (i.e., cTnI and cTnT) are the preferred biomarkers for diagnosing MI. Troponins are proteins found in skeletal and cardiac muscle that attach to tropomyosin. After ischemia, muscle injury, or destruction of muscle, these substances are released into the blood.

For patients presenting with symptoms suggestive of an ACS, practice guidelines recommend obtaining cardiac biomarkers (i.e., troponin levels) on initial presentation and again between 3 and 6 hours later after symptom onset to determine a rising or falling pattern (Amsterdam et al., 2014). The development of high-sensitivity cardiac troponin assays (hs-cTn) has allowed conventional serial biomarker sampling to be shortened to include measurements on initial presentation and 1 to 3 hours later; however, in areas where high-sensitivity assays are not available, serial testing at presentation, and 3 to 6 hours later remains the standard of care (Bonaca & Sabatine, 2022; Gulati et al., 2021).

Fig. **3.7** Progression of myocardial necrosis after coronary artery occlusion. Necrosis begins in a small zone of the myocardium beneath the endocardial surface in the center of the ischemic zone. The area that depends on the occluded vessel for perfusion is the "at risk" myocardium *(shaded)*. Note that a very narrow zone of myocardium immediately beneath the endocardium is spared from necrosis because oxygen and nutrition can be provided by diffusion from the ventricle. (From Kumar, V., Abbas, A. K., & Aster, J. C. [2021]. *Robbins & Cotran pathologic basis of disease* [10th ed.]. Elsevier.)

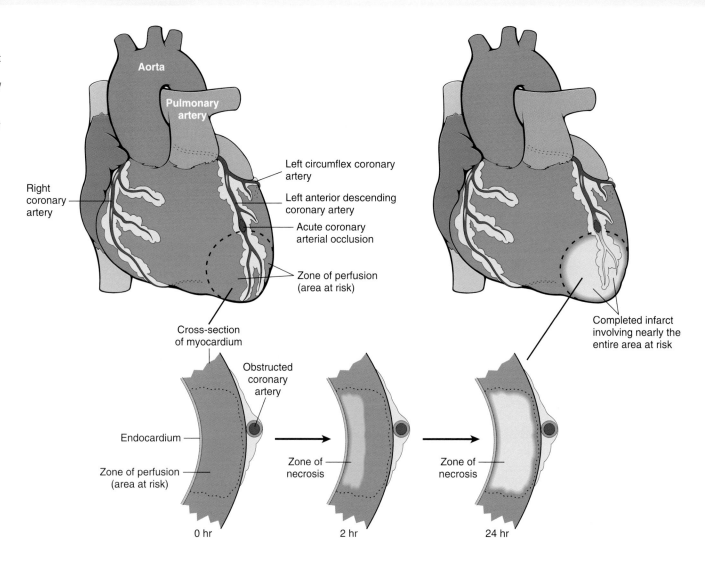

If cardiac biomarkers are absent in the patient's circulation, the diagnosis is UA. If elevated biomarker levels are present (and STE is absent), the diagnosis is NSTEMI. If elevated biomarker levels are present and the ECG shows STE in two or more contiguous leads, the diagnosis is STEMI.

12-Lead ECG

To recognize ECG signs of ischemia, injury, and infarction, you must be able to spot changes in the shape of the QRS complex, ST segment, and T wave. To localize the area at risk, note which leads display that evidence and consider which part of the heart those leads "see." Once the area at risk has been recognized, an understanding of coronary artery anatomy makes it possible to predict which coronary artery is affected. Table 3.1 summarizes the pattern in which coronary arteries most commonly supply the myocardium.

One way to gauge the relative extent of ischemia or infarct size is to evaluate how many leads show indicative changes. For example, an ECG showing changes in only a few leads suggests a smaller affected area than one that produces changes in many leads. In general the more proximal the blockage in the affected vessel, the larger the infarction and the greater the number of leads showing indicative changes.

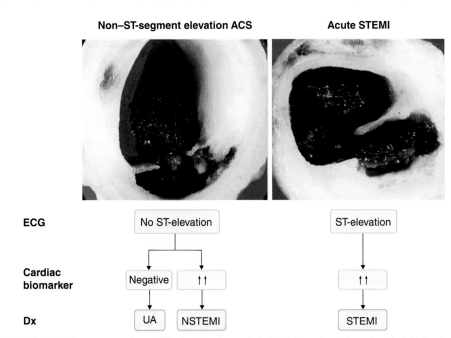

Fig. 3.8 Acute coronary syndrome (ACS). Symptomatic, morphologic, electrocardiographic, and serologic findings in patients with various kinds of ACSs. Individuals with an ACS usually complain of chest pain or discomfort. If the involved coronary artery is totally occluded by fresh thrombus *(right)*, the patient's electrocardiogram (ECG) reveals ST-segment elevation and cardiac biomarkers subsequently are elevated, the patient is diagnosed with an ST-segment elevation myocardial infarction (STEMI). If the involved coronary artery is partially occluded by fresh thrombus *(left)*, the patient's ECG does not show ST-segment elevation. If cardiac biomarkers are not elevated, the patient is diagnosed with unstable angina (UA). If cardiac biomarkers are elevated, the patient is diagnosed with a non-STEMI (NSTEMI). *Dx,*Diagnosis. (From Goldman, L., & Schafer, A. I. [2016]. *Goldman-Cecil medicine* [25th ed.]. Saunders.)

The left ventricle is divided into regions where an MI may occur: the septal, anterior, lateral, inferior, and inferobasal (posterior) (Fig. 3.9). If an ECG shows changes in leads II, III, and aVF, the inferior wall is affected. Because the inferior wall of the left ventricle is supplied by the right coronary artery (RCA) in most people, it is reasonable to suppose that these ECG changes result from partial or complete RCA blockage. When indicative changes are seen in the leads viewing the septal, anterior, and/or lateral walls of the left ventricle (V$_1$ to V$_6$, I, and aVL), it is reasonable to suspect that these ECG changes are the result of partial or complete blockage of the LCA. Locating an MI based on ECG changes is discussed in more detail later in this chapter.

Unstable Angina and Non-ST-Elevation Myocardial Infarction

UA, also known as *preinfarction angina, accelerating* or *crescendo angina, intermediate coronary syndrome*, and *preocclusive syndrome*, is a condition of intermediate severity between stable angina and acute MI. With UA and NSTEMI, partial occlusion of a

TABLE 3.1   Localization of a Myocardial Infarction

Anatomic Region	ECG Changes	Probable Culprit Coronary Artery
Anterior wall	Indicative changes: V$_3$, V$_4$ Reciprocal changes: III, aVF (if antero-lateral MI), V$_7$, V$_8$, V$_9$	LAD
Septum	Indicative changes: V$_1$, V$_2$ Reciprocal changes: V$_7$, V$_8$, V$_9$	LAD
Inferior wall	Indicative changes: II, III, aVF Reciprocal changes: I, aVL	RCA (most common) or Cx
Lateral wall	Indicative changes: I, aVL, V$_5$, V$_6$ Reciprocal changes: III, aVF (if high-lateral MI)	LAD, Cx, or RCA
Right ventricle	Indicative changes: V$_1$R to V$_6$R Reciprocal changes: I, aVL	RCA
Inferobasal (posterior) wall	Indicative changes: V7, V$_8$, V$_9$ Reciprocal changes: V$_1$, V$_2$, V$_3$	RCA or Cx
Diffuse subendocardial ischemia	Indicative changes: aVR, V$_1$ Reciprocal changes: I, II, aVL, V$_4$, V$_5$, V$_6$ (may involve additional leads)	LMCA, proximal LAD, or 3-vessel disease

Cx, Circumflex artery; *ECG,* electrocardiogram; *LAD,* left anterior descending; *LCA,* left coronary artery; *LMCA,* left main coronary artery; *MI,* myocardial infarction; *RCA,* right coronary artery.

coronary artery occurs that limits coronary blood flow, leading to subendocardial ischemia (UA) and possible subendocardial necrosis (NSTEMI) in the area perfused by the affected coronary artery.

12-Lead ECG

UA and NSTEMI are often grouped as non-ST-elevation ACSs (NSTE-ACSs) because ECG changes associated with these conditions usually include ST-segment depression and T-wave inversion in the leads facing the affected area (Figs. 3.10 and 3.11). Experts note that ST-segment depression of 1 mm or more in six leads, which may be associated with STE in leads aVR or lead V1 and hemodynamic compromise, is suggestive evidence of multivessel disease or left main disease (Thygesen et al., 2018).

Consider This

If a patient presents with a possible ACS and the only ST-segment change seen on a standard 12-lead ECG is depression (particularly in leads V$_1$ through V$_4$), strongly consider obtaining posterior chest leads V$_7$ through V$_9$ to assess for a possible inferobasal (i.e., posterior) infarction.

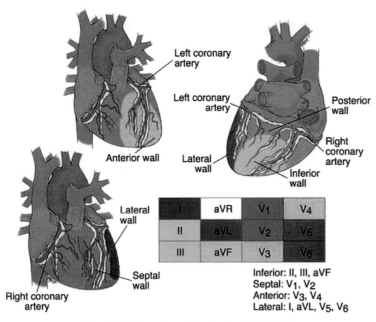

Fig. **3.9** The surfaces of the heart and facing leads.

Inferior: II, III, aVF
Septal: V$_1$, V$_2$
Anterior: V$_3$, V$_4$
Lateral: I, aVL, V$_5$, V$_6$

ST-Elevation Myocardial Infarction

Recall that with NSTE-ACS, a coronary artery is *partially* occluded, which can lead to subendocardial ischemia in the distribution of the affected coronary artery. With STEMI, an epicardial coronary artery is *completely* blocked. This occlusion can result in myocardial ischemia that affects the ventricular wall's entire thickness (i.e., transmural) (see Fig. 3.6).

12-Lead ECG

ECG changes associated with STEMI often occur in a predictable pattern. The ECG changes described here appear in leads looking at the area fed by the blocked (culprit) vessel.

- *Hyperacute T waves*. Within minutes of an interruption of coronary blood flow (usually within the first 30 minutes), hyperacute T waves may be observed on the ECG in the leads facing the affected area. Hyperacute T waves are tall, broad, and peaked and are considered a STEMI equivalent (Kontos et al., 2022) (Fig. 3.12). Clinically, hyperacute T waves may not be observed because these ECG changes may have resolved by the time the patient seeks medical assistance. In addition to acute myocardial ischemia and infarction, possible causes of tall T waves include hyperkalemia, left ventricular hypertrophy, left bundle branch block (BBB), acute pericarditis, acute central nervous system events (e.g., intracranial hemorrhage), and benign early repolarization, among others.

Consider This

Although rarely observed, persistent hyperacute T waves with a preceding J point depression in the chest leads, known as "de Winter's T waves," may be indicative of a complete occlusion of the proximal left anterior descending (LAD) coronary artery (Langowski & Roantree, 2020).

- *ST-segment changes.* Evidence of myocardial injury can be seen on the ECG as STE (Box 3.4, Fig. 3.13). Continuous ST-segment monitoring can help detect ST-segment changes that confirm the diagnosis of an ACS and detect silent or unrecognized myocardial ischemia.

Consider This

Conditions other than STEMI can cause STE. Examples of these conditions include benign early repolarization, pericarditis, BBB, and ventricular-paced rhythms, among others. These conditions are discussed in Chapter 4.

- *QRS changes.* Pathologic Q waves signify abnormal electrical activity (Scirica et al., 2022), are correlated with more extensive myocardial injury (Holicka et al., 2021), and are associated with worsened outcomes. If Q waves develop, they may appear early during an MI or, more commonly, develop 8 to 16 hours after vessel occlusion. An MI was once classified according to its location (e.g., anterior, inferior) and if it produced Q waves on the ECG over several days. A *Q-wave infarction* was considered synonymous with *transmural infarction*, and a *non–Q-wave infarction* was previously termed a *subendocardial infarction*. This terminology has been replaced because a pathologic Q wave may take hours to develop (and, in some cases, never develop) and because cardiac magnetic resonance studies indicate that the development of a Q wave on the ECG is determined more by the size of the infarction than by the depth of mural involvement (Scirica et al., 2022). Q waves may persist after the infarction, decrease in amplitude, or resolve over time.
- *T-wave inversion.* In a patient experiencing an ACS, inverted T waves suggest ischemia. T-wave inversion may precede the development of ST-segment changes, or they may occur simultaneously. T waves associated with ischemia and infarction may remain inverted for varying periods ranging from days, weeks, or months, or they may remain permanently (Wagner et al., 2009).

Localizing a Myocardial Infarction

Leads that view the same surfaces of the heart can be grouped and analyzed for ECG evidence of myocardial ischemia, injury, or infarction. Because ECG evidence must be found in at least two contiguous leads, assessing lead groupings for indicative changes

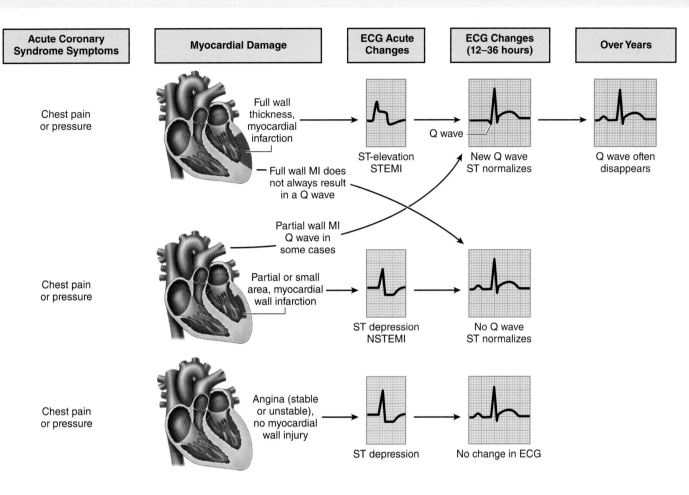

Acute Coronary Syndrome Symptoms	Myocardial Damage	ECG Acute Changes	ECG Changes (12–36 hours)	Over Years

Chest pain or pressure — Full wall thickness, myocardial infarction — ST-elevation STEMI — Q wave — New Q wave ST normalizes — Q wave often disappears

— Full wall MI does not always result in a Q wave

Partial wall MI Q wave in some cases

Chest pain or pressure — Partial or small area, myocardial wall infarction — ST depression NSTEMI — No Q wave ST normalizes

Chest pain or pressure — Angina (stable or unstable), no myocardial wall injury — ST depression — No change in ECG

Fig. **3.10** Acute coronary syndromes: ST-elevation myocardial infarction (STEMI), non–ST-elevation myocardial infarction (NSTEMI), and unstable angina. Electrocardiography changes over time. (From Urden, L. D., Stacy, K. M., & Lough, M. E. [2022]. *Critical care nursing: Diagnosis and management* [9th ed.]. Elsevier.)

helps determine the location of the area at risk and predict which coronary artery is affected. In general, the more proximal the vessel blockage, the larger the infarction and the greater the number of leads showing indicative changes.

Consider This

Factors including the anatomic position and size of the heart, the patient's unique pattern of coronary artery distribution, the location of the occlusion along the length of the coronary artery, the presence of collateral circulation, previous infarctions, and concomitant medication- and electrolyte-related ECG changes may also affect the perceived location of an infarction versus its actual location.

When viewing the 12-lead ECG of a patient experiencing an ACS, look at each lead for ST-segment displacement (i.e., elevation or depression). If ST-segment displacement is present, note its displacement in millimeters. Next, inspect the T waves for any changes in orientation, shape, and size. Finally, examine each lead for the presence of a Q wave. If a Q wave is present, measure its duration.

Anterior Infarction

An anterior infarction occurs when the blood supply to the LAD artery is disrupted (Fig. 3.14). Evidence can be seen in leads V_3 and V_4, which face the anterior wall of the left ventricle. Septal involvement is evidenced by changes in leads V_1 and V_2 (Fig. 3.15). Proximal occlusion of the LAD may become an anteroseptal infarction if the septal branch is involved. ECG changes indicative of an anteroseptal infarction should be visible

Fig. 3.11 Marked ST-segment depression in a patient with prolonged chest pain is the result of an acute non–ST-segment elevation myocardial infarction. Between 1 and 3 mm of ST-segment depression is seen in leads I, aVL, and V_4 to V_6. The patient is known to have had a previous inferior myocardial infarction. (From Andreoli, T. E., Benjamin, I. J., Griggs, R. C., & Wing, E. J. [2010]. *Andreoli and Carpenter's Cecil essentials of medicine.* Saunders.)

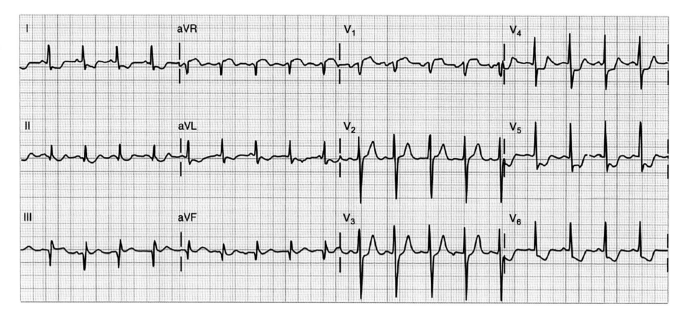

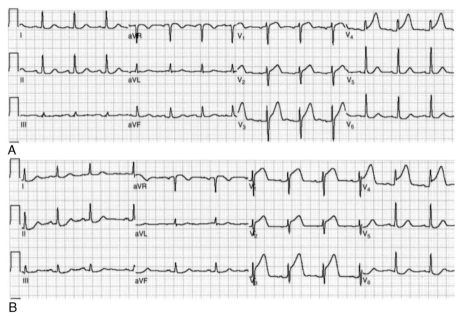

Fig. 3.12 Hyperacute T wave of acute myocardial infarction. (A) Note the broad, tall T waves in leads V_3 and V_4 in this patient with chest pain and diaphoresis. These are the hyperacute T waves of early ST-segment elevation myocardial infarction. The ST segment is just beginning to rise in leads V_3 and V_4; leads V_1 and V_2 are also suspicious. (B) This tracing is from the same patient, roughly 30 minutes after the electrocardiogram in (A). Note the prominent ST-segment elevation in leads V_1 to V_4. (From Walls, R.M., Hockberger, R.S., Gausche-Hill, M., Erickson, T.B., & Wilcox, S.R. [2023]. *Rosen's emergency medicine: Concepts and clinical practice.* [10th ed.]. Elsevier.)

| Box **3.4** | **ST-Segment Elevation** |

In a patient experiencing an ACS, and in the absence of left ventricular hypertrophy and BBB, new or presumed new STE of 1 mm or more at the J point in two or more contiguous leads (other than V_2 and V_3) is suggestive of myocardial injury. STE definitions vary by patient age and sex for leads V_2 and V_3 as follows:

- 2.5 mm or more in men younger than 40 years
- 2 mm or more in men 40 years or older
- 1.5 mm or more in women regardless of age

Data from Thygesen, K., Alpert, J. S., Jaffe, A. S., Chaitman, B. R., Bax, J. J., Morrow, D. A., & White, H. D. Fourth universal definition of myocardial infarction (2018). *Journal of the American College of Cardiology, 72*(18), 2231–2264.

in leads V_1 through V_4 (Fig. 3.16). An anterolateral infarction may result if the marginal branch is involved (Table 3.2).

If the chest leads indicate ECG changes in leads V_3 and V_4 (suggestive of an anterior MI) and indicative changes are also present in V_5 and V_6, the infarction would be called an *anterolateral infarction.* ECG changes with this type of infarction are also possible in leads I and aVL. If the blockage occurs proximal to both the septal and diagonal branches, an extensive anterior infarction (anteroseptal-lateral MI) will result. ECG changes should be visible in leads V_1 through V_6, as well as leads I and aVL. Research shows that STE of 1 mm or more in lead aVR on admission was a strong and independent predictor of major adverse cardiovascular events within 30 days of discharge for patients who experienced an anterior STEMI (Sedighi et al., 2021).

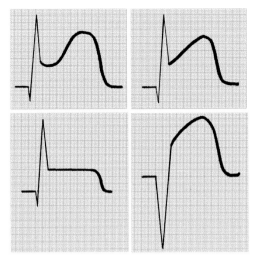

Fig. **3.13** Various shapes of ST-segment elevation seen with acute myocardial infarctions. (From Goldberger, A. L., Goldberger, Z. D., & Shvilkin, A. [2018]. *Goldberger's clinical electrocardiography: A simplified approach* [9th ed.]. Elsevier.)

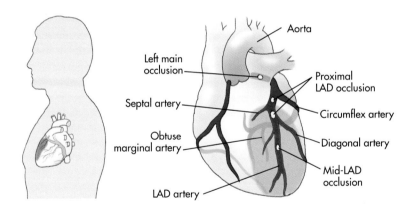

I Lateral	aVR	V₁ Septum	V₄ Anterior
II Inferior	aVL Lateral	V₂ Septum	V₅ Lateral
III Inferior	aVF Inferior	V₃ Anterior	V₆ Lateral

Fig. **3.14** Anterior infarction. Occlusion of the midportion of the left anterior descending (LAD) artery results in an anterior infarction. Proximal occlusion of the LAD may become an anteroseptal infarction if the septal branch is involved or an anterolateral infarction if the marginal branch is involved. An extensive anterior infarction will result if the occlusion occurs proximal to the septal and diagonal branches.

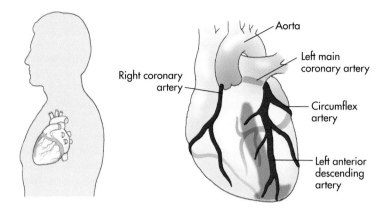

I Lateral	aVR	V₁ Septum	V₄ Anterior
II Inferior	aVL Lateral	V₂ Septum	V₅ Lateral
III Inferior	aVF Inferior	V₃ Anterior	V₆ Lateral

Fig. **3.15** Septal infarction.

Poor R-wave progression is a phrase used to describe R waves that decrease in size from V_1 to V_4. Possible causes include right or left ventricular hypertrophy and left BBB. Poor R-wave progression may also be a nonspecific indicator of anterior wall infarction.

Wellens syndrome is an ECG pattern associated with severe proximal LAD stenosis. Patients with Wellens syndrome typically have a history of chest pain or discomfort. The ECG pattern, which can be transient, is characterized by deeply inverted or biphasic T waves in leads V_2 through V_4, usually during a pain-free period. In addition, there is little or no STE, and cardiac biomarkers may or may not be elevated.

de Winter syndrome, considered an anterior STEMI-equivalent, is associated with acute occlusion of the proximal LAD artery. Patients present with chest pain or discomfort but lack the typical ECG changes of an anterior STEMI. The de Winter ECG pattern includes upsloping ST-segment depression greater than 1 mm at the J point in the chest leads; tall, prominent, and symmetrically peaked T waves with no classic STE in the chest leads; and slight (0.5 to 1 mm) STE in lead aVR (Kontos et al., 2022). With both syndromes, rapid recognition and emergent reperfusion therapy can help avoid the development of an anterior infarction.

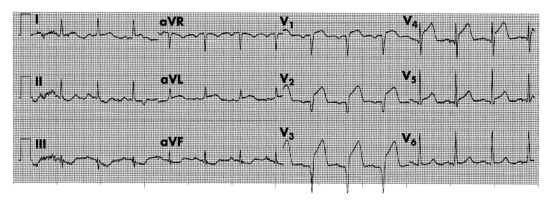

Fig. **3.16** Extensive anteroseptal infarction.

TABLE 3.2	Infarctions Involving the Anterior Wall	
Anatomic Region	**ECG Changes**	**Possible Complications**
Anterior wall	Indicative changes: V_3, V_4 Reciprocal changes: III, aVF (if high lateral MI), V_7, V_8, V_9	Left ventricular dysfunction, including heart failure and cardiogenic shock; AV blocks, BBBs, PVCs, atrial flutter, AFib
Septum	Indicative changes: V_1, V_2 Reciprocal changes: V_7, V_8, V_9	
Anteroseptal	Indicative changes: V_1 to V_4 Reciprocal changes: V_7, V_8, V_9	
Anterolateral	Indicative changes: I, aVL, V_3 to V_6 Reciprocal changes: III, aVF (if high lateral MI), V_7, V_8, V_9	

AFib, Atrial fibrillation; *AV,* atrioventricular; *BBB,* bundle branch block; *MI,* myocardial infarction; *PVC,* premature ventricular complex.

Consider This

Experts observe that although 85% to 90% of STEMI patients experience restored coronary flow with primary percutaneous coronary intervention (PCI), microcirculatory perfusion and myocardial metabolism are not restored in about 50% of cases (Kloner et al., 2021). In 2019, the US Food and Drug Administration approved supersaturated oxygen (SSO_2) therapy for patients with anterior STEMI immediately after successful PCI with stenting within 6 hours of symptom onset. After opening the culprit vessel, hyperoxygenated blood is infused through a small catheter in the left main coronary artery for 60 minutes. This intervention, used as an adjunct to reperfusion therapy, helps resolve endothelial edema, restore microvascular flow, and reperfuse ischemic myocardium and has been shown to reduce infarct size and improve cardiac function.

Inferior Infarction

Leads II, III, and aVF view the inferior surface of the left ventricle. In most individuals, the inferior wall of the left ventricle is supplied by the posterior descending branch of the RCA ("right dominant system"). Blockage of the RCA proximal to the marginal branch will result in an inferior MI and right ventricular infarction (RVI). Blockage of the RCA distal to the marginal branch will result in an inferior infarction, sparing the right ventricle (Fig. 3.17, Table 3.3). Reciprocal changes are observed in leads I and aVL.

In some individuals, the circumflex artery (Cx) supplies the inferior wall through the posterior descending artery ("left dominant system"). Blockage of the posterior descending artery will result in an inferior infarction; however, a proximal occlusion of the Cx may result in infarction in the lateral and posterior walls. STE in lead V_1 in the presence of an inferior STEMI (with elevation greater in lead III than in lead II) suggests associated RVI (Glass III & Brady, 2023). Fig. 3.18 is an example of an acute inferior infarction.

Right Ventricular Infarction

RVI should be suspected when ECG changes suggesting an inferior infarction (STE in leads II, III, and/or aVF) are observed. The right ventricle is supplied by the right ventricular marginal branch of the RCA (Fig. 3.19). Blockage of the right ventricular marginal branch results in an isolated RVI. Blockage of the RCA proximal to the right ventricular marginal branch results in an inferior RVI.

Right chest leads are used to view the right ventricle (Table 3.4). If time does not permit the acquisition of all six right-sided chest leads, the leads of choice are V_3R and V_4R (Wagner et al., 2009). The most sensitive ECG signs of right ventricular injury include 1-mm STE in lead V_1 and in lead V_4R (O'Gara et al., 2013). Be sure to record the right chest leads as quickly as possible after the onset of ACS symptoms because the STE associated with RVI persists for a much shorter period than the STE associated with inferior infarction observed in the limb leads (Wagner et al., 2009). Fig. 3.20 shows an example of RVI.

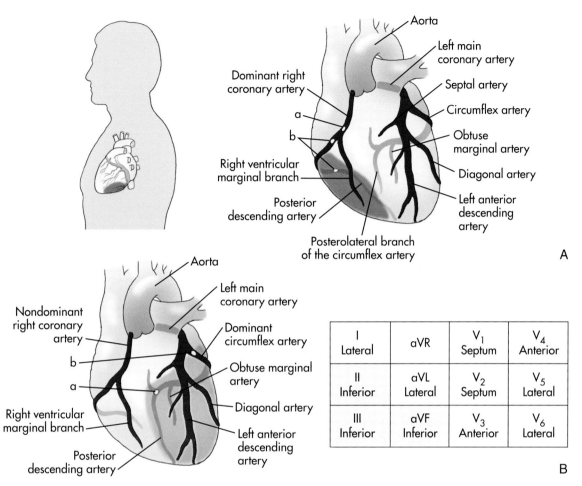

Fig. **3.17** (A) Inferior wall infarction. Coronary anatomy shows a dominant right coronary artery (RCA). A blockage at point "a" results in an inferior infarction and right ventricular infarction. A blockage at point "b" involves only the inferior wall, sparing the right ventricle. (B) Inferior wall infarction. Coronary anatomy shows a dominant circumflex artery. A blockage at point "a" results in an inferior infarction. A blockage at "b" may result in a lateral and inferobasal infarction.

I Lateral	aVR	V$_1$ Septum	V$_4$ Anterior
II Inferior	aVL Lateral	V$_2$ Septum	V$_5$ Lateral
III Inferior	aVF Inferior	V$_3$ Anterior	V$_6$ Lateral

Patients experiencing an inferior STEMI and RVI are at increased risk of sinus arrest/ severe bradycardia, AV block, cardiogenic shock, major adverse cardiovascular events, and major bleeding compared with those without RVI (Hu et al., 2022).

Consider This

It is sometimes possible to detect the presence of RVI by closely examining lead V$_1$. V$_1$ and V$_2$ may occasionally show STE from an RVI because V$_1$ is located in the same position as V$_2$R, and V$_2$ is also V$_1$R. When an inferior infarction exists and the ST segment is elevated in V$_1$ and/or V$_2$, an RVI is presumed to exist when the amount of STE is greater in V$_1$ than in V$_2$. Conversely, when V$_1$ and V$_2$ show STE because of a septal infarction, the amount of STE is typically greater in V$_2$ than in V$_1$. The use of V$_1$ as an indicator for RVI is fairly specific but not very sensitive.

TABLE **3.3**	Inferior Infarction	
Anatomic Region	**ECG Changes**	**Possible Complications**
Inferior wall	Indicative changes: II, III, aVF Reciprocal changes: I, aVL	Bradydysrhythmias; AV blocks

AV, Atrioventricular.

Lateral Infarction

Lateral wall infarctions often occur as extensions of anterior or inferior infarctions because the lateral wall of the left ventricle may be supplied by the Cx, the LAD artery, or a branch of the RCA. Because the lateral wall of the left ventricle is viewed by a combination of chest (V$_5$ and V$_6$) and limb (I and aVL) leads, evidence of a lateral wall infarction may be seen in some or all of the following leads: I, aVL, V$_5$, and V$_6$ (Fig. 3.21, Table 3.5). The

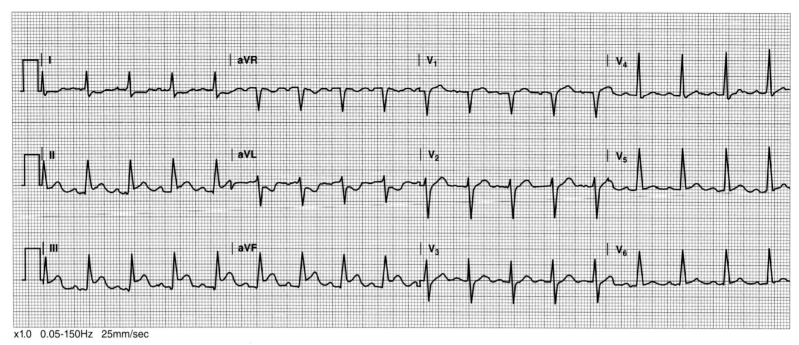

x1.0 0.05-150Hz 25mm/sec

Fig. **3.18** Acute inferior infarction. Note the ST-segment elevation in leads II, III, and aVF and the reciprocal ST depression in leads I and aVL. Abnormal Q waves are also present in leads II, III, and aVF.

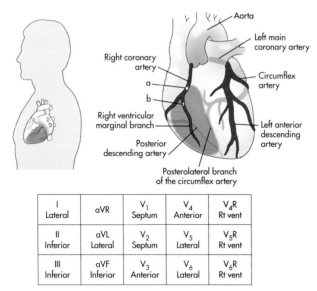

I Lateral	aVR	V$_1$ Septum	V$_4$ Anterior	V$_4$R Rt vent
II Inferior	aVL Lateral	V$_2$ Septum	V$_5$ Lateral	V$_5$R Rt vent
III Inferior	aVF Inferior	V$_3$ Anterior	V$_6$ Lateral	V$_6$R Rt vent

Fig. **3.19** Right ventricular infarction (RVI). At "a," blockage of the right coronary artery proximal to the right ventricular marginal branch results in an inferior and RVI. At "b," blockage of the right ventricular marginal branch results in an isolated RVI.

TABLE **3.4**	Right Ventricular Infarction	
Anatomic Region	**ECG Changes**	**Possible Complications**
Right ventricle	Indicative changes: V$_1$R to V$_6$R Reciprocal changes: I, aVL	Sinus arrest/severe bradycardia, AV blocks, cardiogenic shock, major adverse cardiovascular events, major bleeding
Inferior and RVI	Indicative changes: II, III, aVF, V$_1$R to V$_6$R Reciprocal changes: I, aVL	

AV, Atrioventricular; *RVI,* right ventricular infarction.

term *high lateral infarction* is used to describe ST changes viewed in leads I and aVL. The term *low lateral infarction* is used to describe ST changes viewed in leads V$_5$ and V$_6$. Reciprocal changes of a high lateral infarction can usually be seen in leads II, III, and aVF.

Isolated lateral wall infarctions usually involve occlusion of the Cx and are often missed. More commonly, the lateral wall is involved with proximal occlusion of the LAD (anterolateral MI) or a branch of the RCA (inferolateral MI). An example of a lateral infarction is shown in Fig. 3.22.

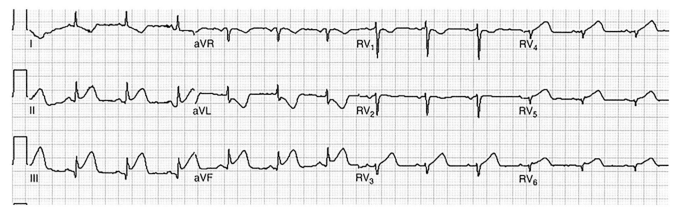

Fig. **3.20** Inferior infarction with right ventricular infarction (RVI). ST-segment elevation (STE) of inferior acute myocardial infarction is present, as is reciprocal ST-segment depression in leads I and aVL. In addition, STE is noted in leads RV_3 to RV_6 (V_3R to V_6R), consistent with RVI. (From Walls, R.M., Hockberger, R.S., Gausche-Hill, M., Erickson, T.B., & Wilcox, S.R. [2023]. *Rosen's emergency medicine: Concepts and clinical practice.* [10th ed.]. Elsevier.)

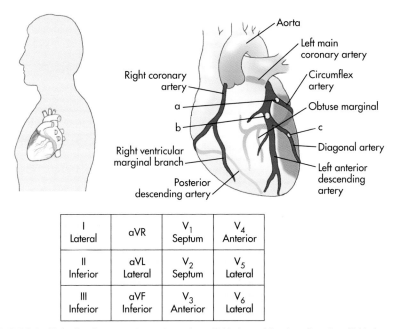

I Lateral	aVR	V_1 Septum	V_4 Anterior
II Inferior	aVL Lateral	V_2 Septum	V_5 Lateral
III Inferior	aVF Inferior	V_3 Anterior	V_6 Lateral

Fig. **3.21** Lateral infarction. Coronary artery anatomy shows (A) blockage of the circumflex artery, (B) blockage of the proximal left anterior descending artery, and (C) blockage of the diagonal artery.

Inferobasal Infarction

Although posterior MIs can occur in isolation, they often occur in conjunction with an inferior or lateral infarction. Experts recommend the term *inferobasal wall* be used instead of *posterior wall*. In most patients, the inferobasal wall of the left ventricle is supplied by the Cx coronary artery; however, it is supplied by the RCA in some patients.

TABLE **3.5**	Lateral Infarction	
Anatomic Region	**ECG Changes**	**Possible Complications**
Lateral wall	Indicative changes: I, aVL, V_5, V_6 Reciprocal changes: II, III, aVF (if high lateral infarction); aVR	Dysrhythmias

Because no leads of a standard 12-lead ECG directly view the inferobasal wall of the left ventricle, additional chest leads (e.g., V_7, V_8, V_9) should be used to view the heart's posterior surface. Indicative changes of an inferobasal infarction include STE of 0.5 mm or more in at least one of these leads (Fig. 3.23, Table 3.6). In addition, R waves larger than S waves in V_2, horizontal (flat) ST-segment depression in V_1 through V_3, and positive T waves in the anterior leads may be seen (Kontos et al., 2022). An example of an inferobasal infarction is shown in Fig. 3.24.

Exceptions

The indicative changes described in this chapter are not absolute, and not every infarction follows this pattern. However, once these indicative changes are understood, they can be applied to individual patient settings and used as a reference point. Several notable exceptions exist to the "classic" pattern of indicative changes.

Indicative changes may occur in a different order or time frame than described. For example, some infarctions do not develop a Q wave, whereas others may lose their Q wave sometime after the infarction. Conversely, some patients' ECGs continue to show persistent STE indefinitely after the infarction.

Other exceptions relate to the localization of the infarction. While ECG localization of the site of infarction is possible, it is not perfect. For example, what appears to be a

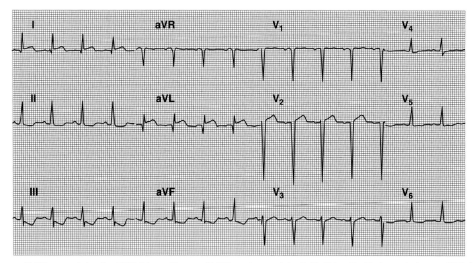

Fig. 3.22 Lateral wall infarction. Lead I shows a small Q wave with ST-segment elevation (STE). A larger Q wave with STE can be seen in lead aVL. This patient had an anterior non–STE infarction four days earlier with STE and T-wave inversion in leads V_2 through V_6. A coronary arteriogram at that time showed a blocked left anterior descending artery distal to its first large septal perforator. The STE evolved and the T waves in all of the chest leads had become upright the day before this tracing was recorded. The patient then had another episode of chest pain associated with the appearance of signs of acute lateral infarction, as shown in this tracing. A repeat coronary arteriogram showed new blockage of the obtuse marginal branch of the circumflex artery. (From Surawicz, B., & Knilans, T. K. [2001]. *Chou's electrocardiography in clinical practice: Adult and pediatric* [5th ed.]. Saunders.)

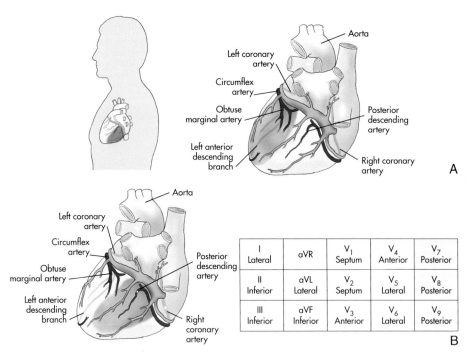

Fig. 3.23 Location of an inferobasal (posterior) infarction. (A) Coronary anatomy shows a dominant right coronary artery (RCA). Occlusion of the RCA commonly results in an inferior and posterior infarction. (B) Coronary anatomy shows a dominant circumflex artery. Occlusion of a marginal branch is the cause of most isolated posterior infarctions.

TABLE **3.6**	Inferobasal (Posterior) Infarction	
Anatomic Region	**Indicative Changes**	**Possible Complications**
Inferobasal	Indicative changes: V_7, V_8, V_9 Reciprocal changes: R waves larger than S waves in V_2, ST depression in V_1 through V_3, positive T waves in anterior leads	SA and AV node dysfunction

AV, Atrioventricular; *SA,* sinoatrial.

lateral wall infarction on the ECG may in fact be an anterior wall infarct. This can occur with any infarct location because the ECG is simply a measurement of the current flow on the patient's skin. In addition, anatomic variations, patient position, the patient's unique pattern of coronary artery distribution, and the presence of collateral circulation may affect the perceived infarct location versus the actual location. For these reasons, you may occasionally encounter infarctions that are difficult to localize into the previously mentioned regions. Two common variations are apical infarctions and inferolateral infarctions.

The apex of the heart is the ventricular area most distal to the atria or the bottom "tip" of the heart. This region consists of anterior wall tissue (supplied by the LCA) and inferior wall tissue (supplied by the RCA). Therefore, depending upon the individual's coronary artery distribution, an RCA occlusion may produce an inferior infarction and affect a portion of the anterior wall. Likewise, an LCA occlusion in some individuals will

Standard 12-Lead ECG   **Left Posterior Leads**

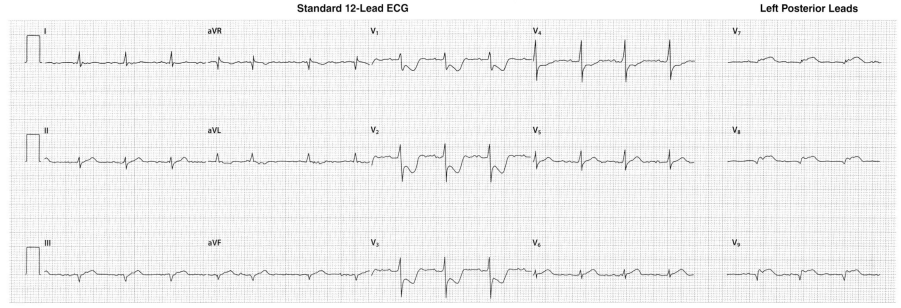

Fig. 3.24 An electrocardiogram recorded in a 76-year-old patient with diabetes during occlusion of the circumflex artery. ST-segment depression is observed in leads V₁ to V₄, which suggests a posterior myocardial infarction (MI). Left posterior leads V₇ to V₉ are helpful in recording ST-segment elevation (STE) that confirms posterior myocardial ischemia. Observing STE in the contiguous posterior leads allows patients with an acute MI to benefit from reperfusion therapy, which would typically be denied based on analysis of the standard 12-lead electrocardiogram alone. (From Wiegand, D. L. [2017]. *AACN procedure manual for high acuity, progressive, and critical care* [7th ed.]. Elsevier.)

affect the anterior wall and extend into the inferior wall. These situations produce what is known as an *apical infarction* (Fig. 3.25).

Another common variation in coronary anatomy distribution may produce an inferolateral infarction. For example, in the portion of the population where the LCA supplies the inferior wall, an occlusion of that artery may produce an infarction involving the inferior and lateral walls. This is one explanation for the inferolateral infarction seen in Fig. 3.26.

Another possible explanation for both apical and inferolateral infarctions is the presence of extensive collateral circulation. In this situation, to some extent, each coronary artery provides blood to tissues generally supplied by the other coronary artery. Therefore, an occlusion in either artery can produce injury in unexpected areas and may produce indicative changes in leads typically supplied by the other coronary artery.

INITIAL MANAGEMENT OF ACUTE CORONARY SYNDROMES

Therapeutic interventions for ACSs aim to improve myocardial tissue oxygen supply, reduce myocardial oxygen demand, protect ischemic myocardium, restore coronary blood flow, preserve left ventricular function, prevent artery reocclusion, and prevent

death. Remember: Time is muscle. As a health care professional, you must recognize an ACS, develop a "working diagnosis" of infarction, and take steps to speed the process of data collection, patient evaluation, and, when appropriate, reperfusion therapy. Early recognition of infarction can significantly reduce *total ischemic time*, which is the time from the onset of STEMI symptoms to successful reperfusion of the blocked coronary artery (O'Gara et al., 2013).

Prehospital Management

When arriving on the scene of a patient complaining of chest discomfort or an anginal equivalent, quickly perform a primary survey and stabilize the patient's airway, breathing, and circulation (ABCs) as necessary. Allow the patient to assume a position of comfort. Ensure the patient does not walk up or down stairs or to the stretcher. Assess vital signs and oxygen saturation. Administer supplemental oxygen if the patient is hypoxemic (SpO₂ below 90%) and titrate therapy to maintain an SpO₂ of 90% or greater (American Heart Association, 2020). In patients with normal oxygen saturation, administering oxygen does not improve symptoms or reduce infarct size, but may result in harm, as evidenced by a larger infarct size on cardiac MRI assessed at six months (Stub et al., 2015).

Obtain a focused history, including the time of symptom onset. Assess and document the patient's pain or discomfort using a 0-to-10 scale. Give chewable non–enteric-coated aspirin as soon as possible if there are no contraindications and establish cardiac

Fig. **3.25** Apical infarction.

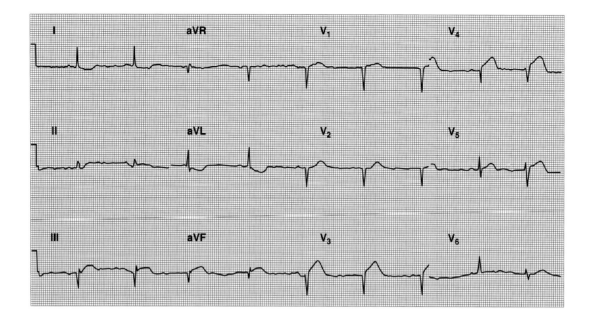

Fig. **3.26** Inferolateral infarction.

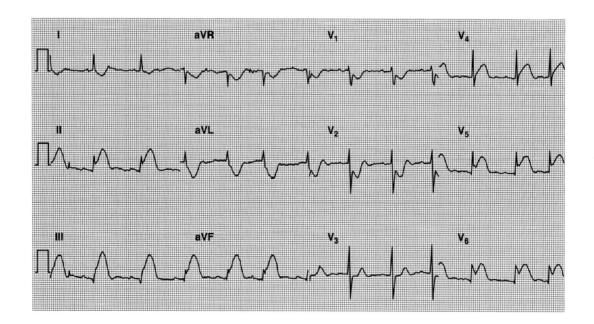

monitoring. Ask the patient about their prescription medications. Determining if the patient is taking beta-blockers, calcium channel blockers, clonidine, digoxin, and/or blood thinners (anticoagulants) will be particularly important to receiving facility staff. Find out if the patient has taken medication for erectile dysfunction or pulmonary hypertension (i.e., a phosphodiesterase inhibitor) within the past 48 hours. Examples include sildenafil (Viagra, Revatio), vardenafil (Levitra, Staxyn), and tadalafil (Cialis, Adcirca). Ask about over-the-counter medicines, herbal supplements, or recreational drugs, such as cocaine, that they may be taking.

Obtain a diagnostic-quality 12-lead ECG within 10 minutes of patient contact for all patients with suspected ACS. Systems of care have been implemented nationwide to improve the quality of care for patients with STEMI. Emergency medical services (EMS) systems, referral and receiving hospitals, emergency physicians, cardiologists, and others work together to minimize total ischemic time. Current guidelines recommend a first medical contact-to-device (FMC2D) time of 90 minutes or less (Kontos et al., 2020).

Three modes of prehospital ECG interpretation exist: (1) interpretation by the paramedic, (2) computerized algorithm interpretation, and (3) ECG transmission for remote interpretation. If transmission capabilities exist, transmit the 12-lead ECG to the emergency physician or cardiologist and determine if the patient meets the criteria for direct transfer to the cardiac catheterization laboratory (CCL). If the patient does not meet the direct-to-CCL transfer criteria, transport the patient to the emergency department (ED) for evaluation. If transmission capabilities do not exist and the 12-lead shows a clear baseline and STE of 1 mm or more in two or more contiguous leads, or if the machine interprets STEMI, notify the ED (Kontos et al., 2020). The patient should be transported to the closest PCI-capable hospital rather than the closest ED if STEMI is confirmed.

Consider This

To reduce reperfusion time when STEMI is identified, the American Heart Association's Mission: Lifeline program recommends EMS activation of the CCL while the patient is en route to the hospital. This recommendation has been poorly adopted because of the frequency of CCL team cancellations after EMS activation, the need to monitor patients until the CCL team arrives, a lack of consensus on direct-to-CCL criteria, and limited resources during off-duty hours (Govea et al., 2021; Kontos et al., 2020).

Perform a secondary assessment during transport as dictated by the patient's condition. Establish intravenous (IV) lines in transit and give medications for pain control per local protocol. For the hemodynamically stable patient experiencing ischemic chest discomfort, up to three doses of sublingual or aerosol NTG can be given at 3- to 5-minute intervals until pain is relieved or hypotension limits its use. Reassess and document the patient's vital signs and level of discomfort after each dose and be prepared to intervene if hypotension occurs. Avoid NTG if the patient has used a phosphodiesterase inhibitor within the past 48 hours.

Morphine sulfate is a potent narcotic analgesic and anxiolytic. In addition, it causes venodilation and can lower heart rate and systolic blood pressure, reducing myocardial oxygen demand. Before giving morphine, assess the degree of the patient's pain or discomfort using a 0-to-10 scale. Reassess and document the patient's vital signs and level of discomfort after each morphine dose. Morphine administration is associated with nausea and vomiting, delayed gastric emptying, decreased intestinal mobility, bradycardia, and respiratory depression. In addition, hypotension may occur, particularly among volume-depleted patients or those who have received vasodilators. Use supine positioning or IV boluses of normal saline (if not contraindicated) to restore blood pressure.

Some clinicians prefer fentanyl (i.e., Sublimaze) for pain relief instead of morphine in patients experiencing an ACS. Fentanyl is a lipid-soluble synthetic opioid with minimal cardiovascular effects and a more rapid onset and shorter duration of action than morphine.

En route, closely monitor the patient for dysrhythmias, hemodynamic instability, and/or the development of cardiogenic shock (e.g., altered mental status, hypotension, cool extremities, tachycardia). Obtain serial 12-lead ECGs, particularly if signs or symptoms change. In addition administering antiarrhythmics, vasopressors, fluid challenges, and/or inotropic agents may be necessary.

Consider This

Some experts recommend avoiding vasodilators, such as NTG, in inferior MI and/or RVI. The rationale for this recommendation is that vasodilators reduce preload, which can potentially cause profound hypotension. However, several studies have observed that infarct location should not preclude nitrate use. For example, in a 2019 study, researchers found that NTG administered for suspected STEMI did not result in a clinically significant decrease in blood pressure compared to patients who did not receive NTG; however, NTG did result in clinically significant pain reduction (Bosson et al., 2019). In addition, a 2021 study found that adverse events associated with pre-hospital NTG administration are more common than previously thought, occurring in about 7% of encounters, but are rare in patients with a systolic blood pressure greater than 110 mm Hg and a heart rate less than 100 beats/min (Popp et al., 2021). These researchers recommended establishing IV access before giving NTG to treat adverse events (e.g., hypotension), should they occur.

Emergency Department Management

Although patients experiencing ischemic chest pain symptoms may arrive in the ED by ambulance, many arrive by private vehicle. Patients who arrive by private vehicle should be triaged immediately. After triage, quickly assess and stabilize the patient's ABCs. Regularly monitor the patient's mental status, vital signs, and oxygen saturation, and perform continuous ECG monitoring. Administer supplemental oxygen if indicated.

If not already done, give aspirin if there are no contraindications, establish IV access, and obtain a portable chest radiograph within 30 minutes. Avoid giving other nonsteroidal antiinflammatory drugs (NSAIDs) because of the increased risk of major adverse cardiac events associated with their use. Obtaining a chest radiograph helps identify high-risk conditions such as pulmonary edema and noncardiac causes for the patient's symptoms; however, do not delay emergent interventions, such as PCI, for those with a definitive STEMI (Kontos et al., 2022). Draw initial laboratory tests, including cardiac biomarkers, electrolytes, and coagulation studies. If the patient is stable, activate the CCL team as soon as STEMI is confirmed.

Obtain a targeted history and physical examination (previously described), which can be done simultaneously with other procedures. Continually reassess the degree of the patient's pain or discomfort using a 0-to-10 scale and reassess the patient's response to medications given. Use risk assessment tools to ascertain the patient's risk of an adverse outcome, determine the need for hospital admission, and make decisions about potential treatment options.

Within 10 minutes of the patient's arrival, carefully review the ECG for evidence of an ACS. Patients experiencing a STEMI are considered the most emergent, followed by those with NSTE-ACS, and then persons experiencing chest pain of probable cardiac origin. Assess the areas of ischemia or injury by assessing lead groupings. Remember: ECG evidence must be found in at least two contiguous leads. If the patient is stable, activate the CCL team as soon as STEMI is confirmed. Stabilize patients experiencing respiratory distress or who are hemodynamically unstable before transport to the CCL.

> **Consider This**
>
> Obtaining and reviewing a 12-lead ECG is an essential component of assessing and managing the patient presenting with ischemic chest discomfort. Obtain the first 12-lead ECG within 10 minutes of patient arrival. Repeat the 12-lead ECG when clinically indicated.

Categorize the patient into one of three groups based on their 12-lead ECG findings: (1) STE, (2) ST-segment depression, or (3) normal/nondiagnostic ECG.

1. **STE**. Patients with STE in two or more contiguous leads are classified as having a STEMI. If STE is seen in leads II, III, and/or aVF, assess the patient for a possible RVI. Because of the urgency for reperfusion in patients with STEMI, providers should not wait for biomarker results to begin treatment; clinical assessment and 12-lead ECG findings should be used to determine initial treatment strategies (Scirica et al., 2022). In addition, current STEMI treatment guidelines and algorithms should be used to guide management decisions, including using pharmacologic reperfusion (i.e., fibrinolytics) or mechanical reperfusion (i.e., PCI) and medical therapies such as antianginal, antiplatelet, and anticoagulant agents; beta-blockers; angiotensin-converting enzyme inhibitors; and statins. Primary PCI is the preferred reperfusion strategy for most patients experiencing STEMI because it is associated with lower rates of recurrent MI, stroke, and death (Atwood, 2022). Once stabilized, emergent PCI should be performed for resuscitated cardiac arrest patients with STE on their ECG (Panchal et al., 2020).

2. **ST-segment depression**. ST depression or transient ST-segment/T-wave changes that occur with pain or discomfort suggest myocardial ischemia. Patients with obvious ST depression in leads V_1 and V_2 should be evaluated for possible inferobasal MI. Current NSTE-ACS guidelines should be used to guide management decisions for these patients.

3. **Normal/nondiagnostic ECG**. A normal ECG or nonspecific ST- and T-wave changes are nondiagnostic and should prompt consideration for further evaluation. Because a normal ECG may be associated with Cx or RCA occlusions and posterior wall ischemia, experts recommend obtaining right-sided ECG leads when such lesions are suspected (Gulati et al., 2021). Compare the ECG obtained with previous ECGs, if available. If symptoms persist and the initial ECG is nondiagnostic, repeat the ECG at 15 to 30-minute intervals during the first hour. Obtain additional ECGs if symptoms persist or change or if troponins are positive.

REFERENCES

American Heart Association. (2020). *2020 Handbook of emergency cardiovascular care for healthcare providers*. American Heart Association.

Amsterdam, E. A., Wenger, N. K., Brindis, R. G., Casey, Jr., D. E., Ganiats, T. G., Holmes, Jr., D. R., Jaffe, A. S., Jneid, H., Kelly, R. F., Kontos, M. C., Levine, G. N., Liebson, P. R., Mukherjee, D., Peterson, E. D., Sabatine, M. S., Smalling, R. W., Zieman, S. J. (2014). 2014 ACC/AHA guideline for the management of patients with non–ST-elevation acute coronary syndromes: A report of the American College of Cardiology/American Heart Association Task Force on Practice Guidelines. *Journal of the American College of Cardiology, 64*(24), 1–150.

Atwood, J. (2022). Management of acute coronary syndrome. *Emergency Medicine Clinics of North America, 40*(4), 693–706.

Bonaca, M. P., & Sabatine, M. S. (2022). Approach to the patient with chest pain. In P. Libby, R. O. Bonow, D. L. Mann, G. F. Tomaselli, D. L. Bhatt, & S. D. Solomon (Eds.), *Braunwald's heart disease: A textbook of cardiovascular medicine* (12th ed., pp. 599–608). Elsevier.

Bosson, N., Isakson, B., Morgan, J. A., Kaji, A. H., Uner, A., Hurley, K., & Niemann, J. T. (2019). Safety and effectiveness of field nitroglycerin in patients with suspected ST-elevation myocardial infarction. *Prehospital Emergency Care, 23*(5), 603–611.

Brown, R. M. (2022). Acute coronary syndrome in women. *Emergency Medicine Clinics of North America, 40*(4), 629–636.

Chen, C., Wei, J., AlBadri, A., Zarrini, P., & Bairey Merz, C. N. (2016). Coronary microvascular dysfunction: Epidemiology, pathogenesis, prognosis, diagnosis, risk factors and therapy. *Circulation Journal, 81*(1), 3–11.

Costello, B. T., & Younis, G. A. (2020). Acute coronary syndrome in women: An overview. *Texas Heart Institute Journal, 47*(2), 128–129.

Damjanov, I. (2017). The cardiovascular system. In *Pathology for the health professions* (5th ed., pp. 133–164). Elsevier.

Glass III, G. F., & Brady, W. J. (2023). Acute coronary syndromes. In R. M. Walls (Ed.), *Rosen's emergency medicine: Concepts and clinical practice* (10th ed., pp. 849–889). Elsevier.

Glickman, S. W., Shofer, F. S., Wu, M. C., Scholer, M. J., Ndubuizu, A., Peterson, E. D., ..., Glickman, L. T. (2012). Development and validation of a prioritization rule for obtaining an immediate 12-lead electrocardiogram in the emergency department to identify ST-elevation myocardial infarction. *American Heart Journal, 163*(3), 372–382.

Govea, A., Lipinksi, J., & Patel, M. P. (2021). Prehospital evaluation, ED management, transfers, and management of inpatient STEMI. *Interventional Cardiology Clinics, 10*(3), 293–306.

Gulati, M., Levy, P. D., Mukherjee, D., Amsterdam, E., Bhatt, D. L., Birtcher, K. K., & Shaw, L. J. (2021). 2021 AHA/ACC/ASE/CHEST/SAEM/SCCT/SCMR guideline for the evaluation and diagnosis of chest pain. *Journal of the American College of Cardiology, 78*(22), e187–e285.

Holicka, M., Cuckova, P., Hnatkova, K., Koc, L., Ondrus, T., Lokaj, P., ..., Malik, M. (2021). In comparison to pathological Q waves, Selvester score is a superior diagnostic indicator of increased long-term mortality risk in ST-elevation myocardial infarction patients treated with primary coronary intervention. *Diagnostics, 11*(5), 799.

Hu, M., Lu, Y., Wan, S., Li, B., Gao, X., Yang, J., ..., Yang, Y. (2022). Long-term outcomes in inferior ST-segment elevation myocardial infarction patients with right ventricular myocardial infarction. *International Journal of Cardiology, 351*, 1–7. doi:10.1016/j.ijcard.2022.01.003.

Kaski, J. C., & Arroyo-Espliguero, R. (2010). Variant angina pectoris. In M. H. Crawford, J. P. DiMarco, & W. J. Paulus (Eds.), *Cardiology* (3rd ed., pp. 301–309). Elsevier.

Kloner, R. A., Creech, J. L., Stone, G. W., O'Neill, W. W., Burkhoff, D., & Spears, J. R. (2021). Update on cardioprotective strategies for STEMI: Focus on supersaturated oxygen delivery. *JACC Basic Translational Science, 6*(12), 1021–1033.

Kontos, M. C., de Lemos, J. A., Deitelzweig, S. B., Diercks, D. B., Gore, M. O., Hess, E. P., ..., Wright, L. J. (2022). 2022 ACC expert consensus decision pathway on the evaluation and disposition of acute chest pain in the emergency department: A report of the American College of Cardiology solution set oversight committee. *Journal of the American College of Cardiology, 80*(20), 1925–1960.

Kontos, M. C., Gunderson, M. R., Zegre-Hemsey, J. K., Lange, D. C., French, W. J., Henry, T. D., ..., Garvey, J. L. (2020). Prehospital activation of hospital resources (PreAct) ST-segment–elevation myocardial infarction (STEMI): A standardized approach to prehospital activation and direct to the catheterization laboratory for STEMI. *Journal of the American Heart Association, 9*(2), e011963.

Lange, R. A., & Hillis, L. D. (2016). Acute coronary syndrome: Unstable angina and non-ST elevation myocardial infarction. In L. Goldman & A. I. Schafer (Eds.), *Goldman-Cecil medicine* (25th ed., pp. 432–441). Saunders.

Langowski, M., & Roantree, R. A. (2020). Hyperacute T waves: An ominous electrocardiogram sign of early myocardial infarction. *Visual Journal of Emergency Medicine, 20*(19), 100747.

Magidson, P. D. (2022). The aged heart. *Emergency Medicine Clinics of North America, 40*(4), 637–649.

Mitchell, R. N., & Connolly, A. J. (2021). The heart. In V. Kumar, A. K. Abbas, & J. C. Aster (Eds.), *Robbins & Cotran pathologic basis of disease* (10th ed., pp. 527–582). Elsevier.

Morrow, D. A., & de Lemos, J. (2022). Stable ischemic heart disease. In P. Libby, R. O. Bonow, D. L. Mann, G. F. Tomaselli, D. L. Bhatt, & S. D. Solomon (Eds.), *Braunwald's heart disease: A textbook of cardiovascular medicine* (12th ed., pp. 739–785). Elsevier.

O'Gara, P. T., Kushner, F. G., Ascheim, D. D., Casey, D. E., Jr., Chung, M. K., de Lemos, J. A., ..., Zhao, D. X. (2013). 2013 ACCF/AHA guideline for the management of ST-elevation myocardial infarction. *Journal of the American College of Cardiology, 61*(4), e78–e140.

Panchal, A. R., Bartos, J. A., Cabañas, J. G., Donnino, M. W., Drennan, I. R., Hirsch, K. G., ..., Berg, K. M. (2020). Part 3: Adult basic and advanced life support: 2020 American Heart Association guidelines for cardiopulmonary resuscitation and emergency cardiovascular care. *Circulation, 142*(16 suppl. 2), S366–S468.

Popp, L. M., Lowell, L. M., Ashburn, N. P., & Stopyra, J. P. (2021). Adverse events after prehospital nitroglycerin administration in a nationwide registry analysis. *American Journal of Emergency Medicine, 50*, 196–201.

Scirica, B. M., Libby, P., & Morrow, D. A. (2022). ST-elevation myocardial infarction: Pathophysiology and clinical evolution. In P. Libby, R. O. Bonow, D. L. Mann, G. F. Tomaselli, D. L. Bhatt, & S. D. Solomon (Eds.), *Braunwald's heart disease: A textbook of cardiovascular medicine* (12th ed., pp. 636–661). Elsevier.

Sedighi, S., Fattahi, M., Dehghani, P., Aslani, A., Mehdipour Namdar, Z., & Hassanzadeh, M. (2021). aVR ST-segment changes and prognosis of ST-segment elevation myocardial infarction. *Health Science Reports, 4*(4), e387. doi:10.1002/hsr2.387.

Stub, D., Smith, K., Bernard, S., Nehme, Z., Stephenson, M., .Bray, J. E., ... on behalf of the AVOID investigators. (2015). Air versus oxygen in ST-segment elevation myocardial infarction. *Circulation, 131*(24), 2143–2150.

Thygesen, K., Alpert, J. S., Jaffe, A. S., Chaitman, B. R., Bax, J. J., Morrow, D. A., & White, H. D. (2018). Fourth universal definition of myocardial infarction. *Journal of the American College of Cardiology, 72*(18), 2231–2264.

Wagner, G. S., Macfarlane, P., Wellens, H., Josephson, M., Gorgels, A., Mirvis, D. M., ..., Gettes, L. S. (2009). AHA/ACCF/HRS recommendations for the standardization and interpretation of the electrocardiogram: Part VI: Acute ischemia/infarction; a scientific statement from the American Heart Association Electrocardiography and Arrhythmias Committee. *Journal of the American College of Cardiology, 53*(11), 1003–1011.

Identify one or more choices that best complete the statement or answer the question.

1. An ACS is usually caused by
   a. hypertension.
   b. coronary artery spasm.
   c. atherosclerotic plaque rupture or erosion.
   d. the inability of the coronary microvasculature to dilate.

2. Vasospastic angina (VA)
   a. is also called microvascular angina.
   b. is caused by spasms of one or more epicardial coronary arteries.
   c. usually produces STE during anginal episodes.
   d. typically occurs in women, individuals with hypertension, and individuals with diabetes.

3. Incomplete occlusion of a coronary artery by a thrombus may result in which of the following?
   a. Sudden death
   b. UA
   c. No clinical signs and symptoms
   d. STEMI
   e. NSTEMI

4. Which of the following patient groups are most likely to present atypically with an ACS?
   a. Older adults
   b. Individuals with diabetes
   c. People assigned female at birth
   d. Patients with a sedentary lifestyle
   e. Middle-aged individuals assigned male at birth
   f. Patients with a family history positive for CAD

5. Supplemental oxygen should be administered
   a. if the SpO_2 value is below 90%.
   b. to all patients experiencing an ACS.
   c. only if STEMI is confirmed via 12-lead ECG.
   d. only if the patient complains of chest discomfort.

6. A 65-year-old man presents with a chief complaint of crushing substernal chest pain that has been present for the past 40 minutes. You should obtain the first 12-lead ECG
   a. within 10 minutes of patient contact.
   b. only after establishing vascular access.
   c. after obtaining biomarkers and a chest radiograph.
   d. if the patient's discomfort persists for more than 30 minutes.
   e. only after administering medications to relieve the patient's discomfort.

7. Which of the following ECG changes is one of the earliest to occur during an infarction, but may have resolved by the time the patient seeks medical assistance?
   a. Pathologic Q waves
   b. Hyperacute T waves
   c. Horizontal ST-segments
   d. Lengthening of the QT interval

8. In a patient experiencing an ACS, inverted T waves suggest the presence of
   a. injury.
   b. ischemia.
   c. infarction.
   d. cardiogenic shock.

9. A patient has been diagnosed with an extensive anterior STEMI. When examining this patient's 12-lead ECG, you should expect to see indicative ECG changes in which of the following leads?
   a. I and aVL
   b. V_7 through V_9
   c. V_1 through V_6
   d. II, III, and aVF
   e. V_1 through V_4, and V_4R

10. Reciprocal changes of a high lateral infarction can usually be viewed in leads
    a. II and aVR.
    b. V_1 through V_3.
    c. V_2 through V_4.
    d. II, III, and aVF.

11. A 66-year-old man is experiencing chest discomfort that he rates 9/10. His 12-lead ECG reveals STE in leads II, III, and aVF and ST-segment depression in leads I and aVL. These ECG findings suggest which of the following?
    a. An inferior STEMI is present.
    b. A posterior STEMI is present
    c. A lateral NSTE-ACS is present.
    d. An anterior NSTE-ACS is present.
    e. The STE reflects reciprocal changes.
    f. The ST-segment depression reflects reciprocal changes.

PRACTICE ECGs

A variety of 12-lead ECGs have been included for practice to help you master the concepts introduced in this chapter (see Figs. 3.27 through 3.35). We recommend the following approach when reviewing a 12-lead ECG:

1. **Identify the rate and underlying rhythm.** Determining rate and rhythm is a priority when interpreting the ECG. If baseline wander or artifact is present to any significant degree, note it. If either of these conditions interferes with the assessment of any lead, use a modifier such as "possible" or "apparent" in your interpretation.
2. **Analyze waveforms, segments, and intervals.** Select one good representative waveform or complex in each lead. Each lead, except for aVR, should be examined for indicative changes, with particular emphasis on ST-segment displacement (elevation or depression). If displacement is present, express it in millimeters. Examine the T waves for any changes in orientation, shape, and size. Note the presence of tall, peaked T waves or T-wave inversion. Examine all leads for pathologic Q waves, which are abnormally wide and deep. Suspect an infarction when Q waves appear in several leads or lead groups, are more than 0.04 second, or are associated with ST or T-wave changes in the same leads (Thygesen et al., 2018).

3. **Examine for evidence of an ACS.** If ST-segment displacement is present, assess the areas of ischemia or injury by evaluating lead groupings. If an ACS is suspected, mentally picture the cardiac anatomy to localize the area at risk and predict which coronary artery is occluded.
4. **Estimate the QRS axis.** Using leads I and aVF, estimate the QRS axis.
5. **Interpret your findings.** Based on your examination, categorize the 12-lead ECG into one of the previously described groups: (1) STE, (2) ST-segment depression, or (3) normal or nondiagnostic ECG.

Our interpretation of each ECG is included at the end of this chapter. Please note that the interpretation of each lead and tracing includes only the material discussed in this text. Therefore, experienced electrocardiographers will note the presence of some conditions or findings that are not listed in the interpretation.

Fig. **3.27**

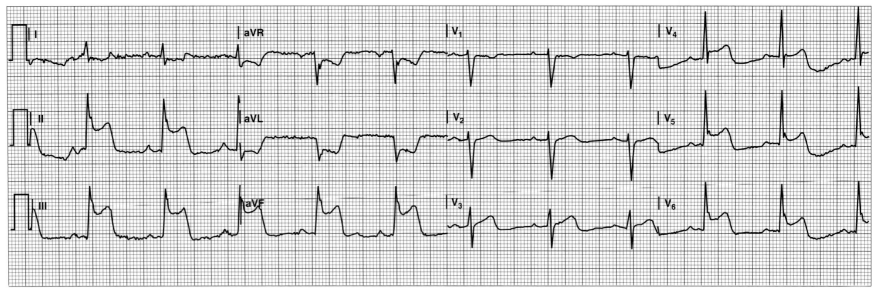

x1.0 0.05-40Hz 25mm/sec

I	Lateral	aVR	---------	V₁	Septum	V₄	Anterior
II	Inferior	aVL	Lateral	V₂	Septum	V₅	Lateral
III	Inferior	aVF	Inferior	V₃	Anterior	V₆	Lateral

Rate and rhythm? _____ STE? _____ ST depression? _____

T-wave changes? _____ Pathologic Q waves? _____ Axis? _____

Interpretation: _____

Fig. **3.28**

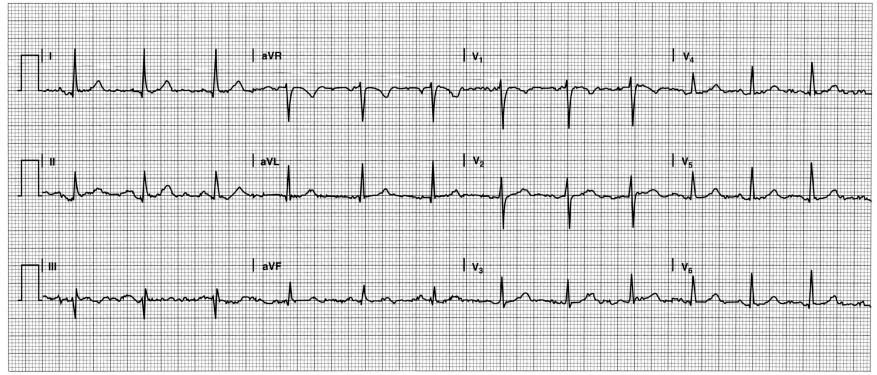

x1.0 0.05-150Hz   25mm/sec

I	Lateral	aVR	---------	V₁	Septum	V₄	Anterior
II	Inferior	aVL	Lateral	V₂	Septum	V₅	Lateral
III	Inferior	aVF	Inferior	V₃	Anterior	V₆	Lateral

Rate and rhythm? _____ STE? _____ ST depression? _____

T-wave changes? _____ Pathologic Q waves? _____ Axis? _____

Interpretation: _____

Fig. **3.29**

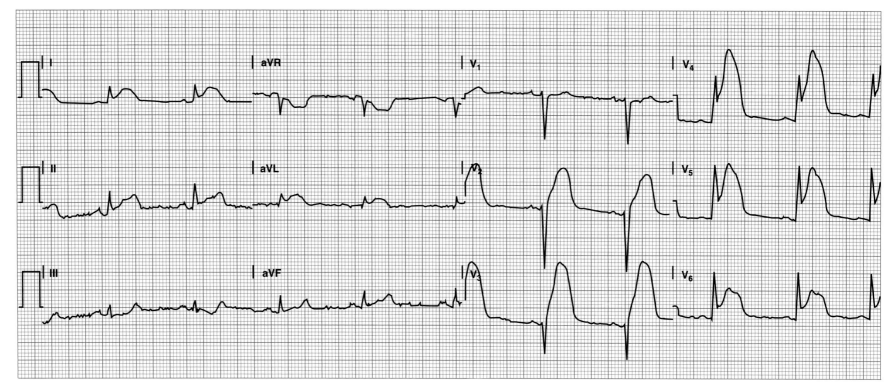

x1.0 0.05-150Hz 25mm/sec

I	Lateral	aVR	---------	V₁	Septum	V₄	Anterior
II	Inferior	aVL	Lateral	V₂	Septum	V₅	Lateral
III	Inferior	aVF	Inferior	V₃	Anterior	V₆	Lateral

Rate and rhythm? _____ STE? _____ ST depression? _____

T-wave changes? _____ Pathologic Q waves? _____ Axis? _____

Interpretation: _____

Fig. **3.30**

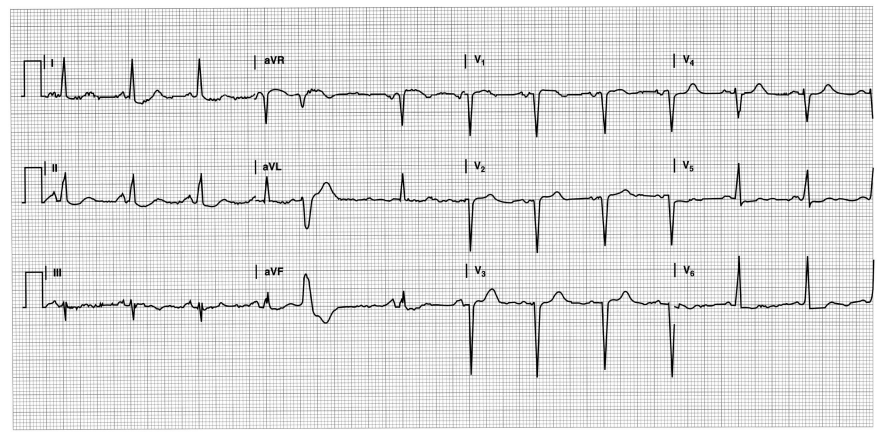

x1.0 0.05-150Hz   25mm/sec

I	Lateral	aVR	---------	V$_1$	Septum	V$_4$	Anterior
II	Inferior	aVL	Lateral	V$_2$	Septum	V$_5$	Lateral
III	Inferior	aVF	Inferior	V$_3$	Anterior	V$_6$	Lateral

Rate and rhythm? _____ STE? _____ ST depression? _____

T-wave changes? _____ Pathologic Q waves? _____ Axis? _____

Interpretation: _____

Fig. **3.31**

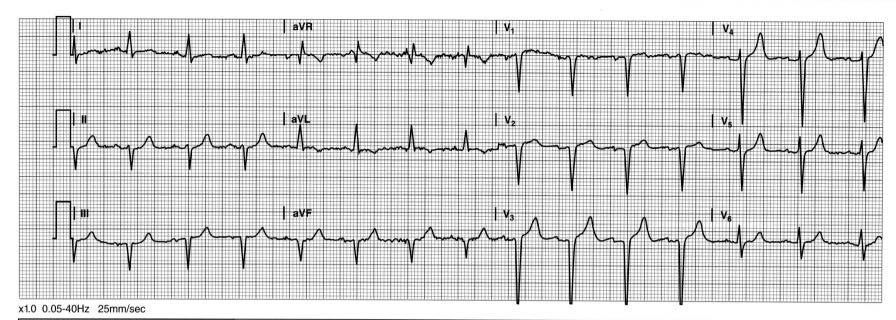

x1.0 0.05-40Hz 25mm/sec

I	Lateral	aVR	---------	V₁	Septum	V₄	Anterior
II	Inferior	aVL	Lateral	V₂	Septum	V₅	Lateral
III	Inferior	aVF	Inferior	V₃	Anterior	V₆	Lateral

Rate and rhythm? _____ STE? _____ ST depression? _____

T-wave changes? _____ Pathologic Q waves? _____ Axis? _____

Interpretation: _____

Fig. **3.32**

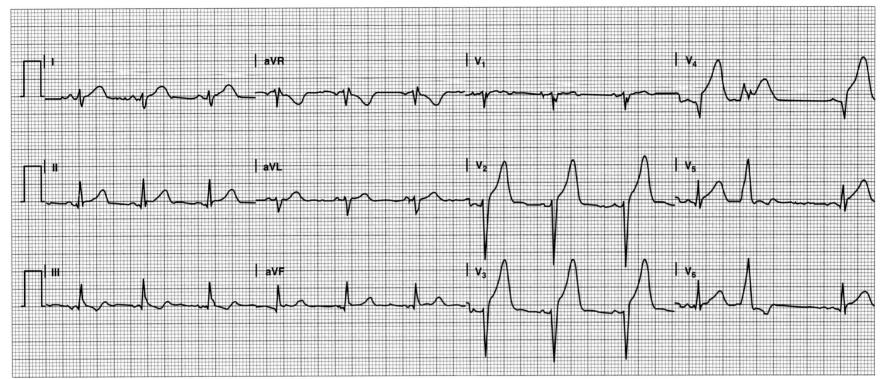

x1.0 0.05-150Hz 25mm/sec

I	Lateral	aVR	---------	V$_1$	Septum	V$_4$	Anterior
II	Inferior	aVL	Lateral	V$_2$	Septum	V$_5$	Lateral
III	Inferior	aVF	Inferior	V$_3$	Anterior	V$_6$	Lateral

Rate and rhythm? _____ STE? _____ ST depression? _____

T-wave changes? _____ Pathologic Q waves? _____ Axis? _____

Interpretation: _____

Fig. 3.33

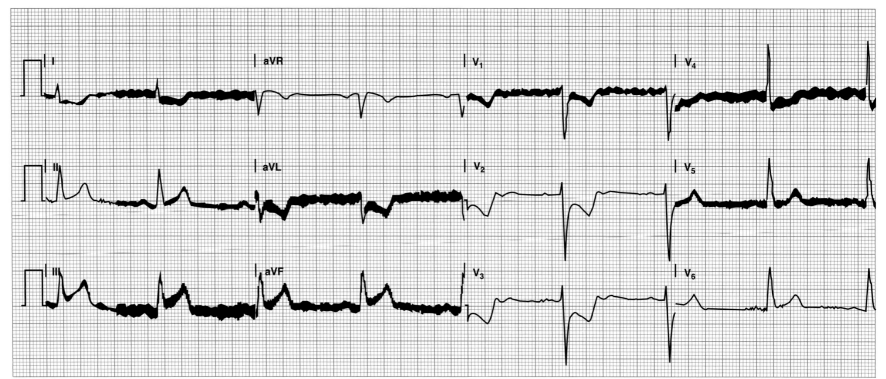

x1.0 0.05-150Hz   25mm/sec

I	Lateral	aVR	---------	V$_1$	Septum	V$_4$	Anterior
II	Inferior	aVL	Lateral	V$_2$	Septum	V$_5$	Lateral
III	Inferior	aVF	Inferior	V$_3$	Anterior	V$_6$	Lateral

Rate and rhythm? _____ STE? _____ ST depression? _____

T-wave changes? _____ Pathologic Q waves? _____ Axis? _____

Interpretation: _____

Fig. **3.34**

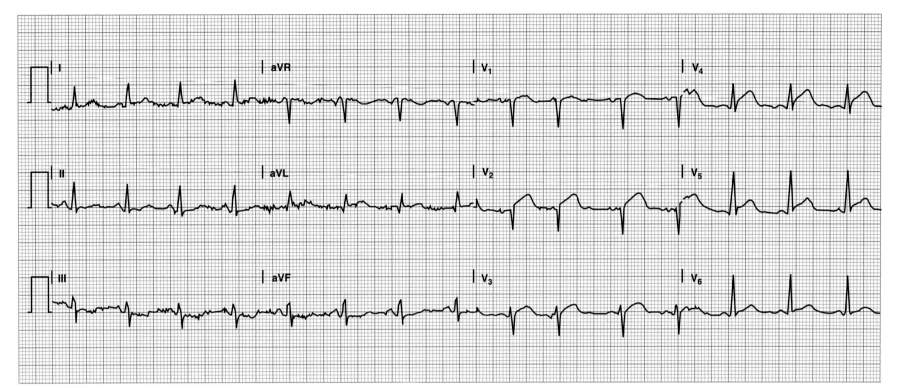

x1.0 0.05-150Hz 25mm/sec

I	Lateral	aVR	---------	V₁	Septum	V₄	Anterior
II	Inferior	aVL	Lateral	V₂	Septum	V₅	Lateral
III	Inferior	aVF	Inferior	V₃	Anterior	V₆	Lateral

Rate and rhythm? _____ STE? _____ ST depression? _____

T-wave changes? _____ Pathologic Q waves? _____ Axis? _____

Interpretation: _____

Fig. **3.35**

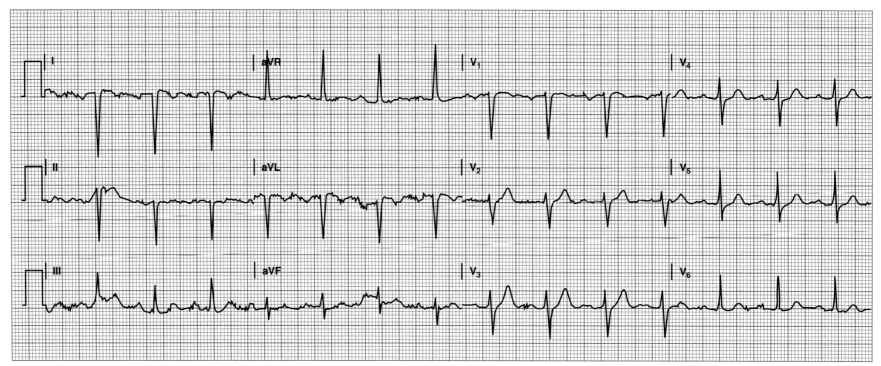

x1.0 0.05-150Hz 25mm/sec

I	Lateral	aVR	---------	V$_1$	Septum	V$_4$	Anterior
II	Inferior	aVL	Lateral	V$_2$	Septum	V$_5$	Lateral
III	Inferior	aVF	Inferior	V$_3$	Anterior	V$_6$	Lateral

Rate and rhythm? _____ STE? _____ ST depression? _____

T-wave changes? _____ Pathologic Q waves? _____ Axis? _____

Interpretation: _____

CASE STUDIES

For each of the following case studies, carefully evaluate the description of the patient's clinical presentation, systematically analyze each 12-lead ECG, and formulate a treatment plan based on the information provided.

CASE STUDY 3.1

A 51-year-old woman presents with a sudden onset of shortness of breath, fatigue, and tingling in her left hand. She denies chest pain or discomfort. The patient reports that she was outside gardening when her symptoms began about 2 hours ago. She has no significant medical history and has no known medication allergies. Her medications include a baby aspirin and a multivitamin daily, as well as melatonin, which she uses as a sleep aide.

Physical examination reveals that the patient is alert and oriented to person, place, time, and event. Her skin is pink, warm, and dry, and her breath sounds are clear. Her SpO_2 is 96% on room air, blood pressure is 128/58 mm Hg, pulse 68 beats/min, and ventilations 18/min. The patient has been placed on a cardiac monitor. Vascular access has been established and a 12-lead ECG has been obtained (Fig. 3.36). Review the patient's ECG and describe your initial interventions for this patient.

Fig. **3.36**

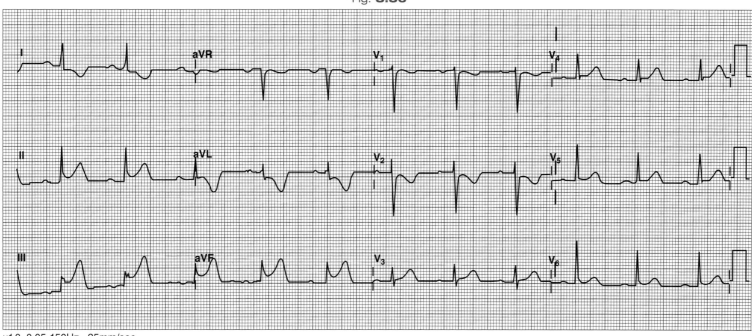

x1.0 0.05-150Hz 25mm/sec

CASE STUDY 3.2

A 58-year-old man presents with crushing substernal chest pain with radiation to his left arm that he rates 10/10. He denies nausea, vomiting, and shortness of breath. The patient states he was putting away dishes when his symptoms began about 45 minutes ago. He has a history of asthma and had a pulmonary embolism 1 year ago, at which time an inferior vena cava umbrella filter was surgically placed. Current medications include warfarin and albuterol. He is allergic to penicillin.

Physical examination reveals the patient is alert and oriented to person, place, time, and event. His skin is pink, warm, and moist; his breath sounds are clear. His SpO$_2$ is 98% on room air, blood pressure is 130/70 mm Hg, pulse 53 beats/min, and ventilations 20/min. The patient has been placed on a cardiac monitor. Vascular access has been established and a 12-lead ECG has been obtained (Fig. 3.37). Review the patient's ECG and describe your initial interventions for this patient.

Fig. **3.37**

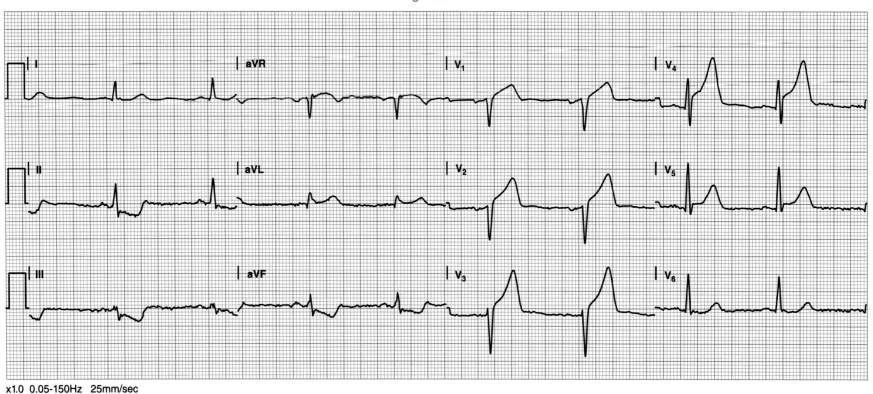

x1.0 0.05-150Hz 25mm/sec

ANSWERS

1. **C.** An ACS is usually caused by atherosclerotic plaque rupture or erosion and thrombus formation leading to reduced coronary artery blood flow and distal myocardial ischemia.

2. **B, C.** Vasospastic agina (VA), also called *Prinzmetal angina* or *Prinzmetal variant angina*, is a form of angina caused by spasms of one or more epicardial coronary arteries. Whereas ECG changes observed with classic angina include ST-segment depression, VA usually produces STE during anginal episodes. Patients with VA are generally younger and have fewer coronary risk factors (except for smoking) than patients with stable angina.

3. **A, B, C, E.** If a coronary artery obstruction is partial or intermittent, the patient may experience no signs and symptoms (i.e., silent ischemia), UA, NSTEMI, or, possibly, sudden death.

4. **A, B, C.** Anginal equivalents are common, particularly in older adults, individuals with diabetes, and people assigned female at birth.

5. **A.** For patients experiencing an ACS, administer supplemental oxygen if the patient is hypoxemic (SpO$_2$ below 90%) and titrate therapy to maintain an SpO$_2$ of 90% or greater.

6. **A.** The 12-lead ECG is an essential diagnostic tool for patients presenting with ischemic chest discomfort or anginal equivalent symptoms. The first 12-lead ECG should be obtained and interpreted within 10 minutes of patient contact. Obtain a repeat 12-lead ECG when clinically indicated by a change in patient condition.

7. **B.** Within minutes of an interruption of coronary blood flow (usually within the first 30 minutes), hyperacute T waves may be observed on the ECG in the leads facing the affected area. Clinically, hyperacute T waves may not be observed because these ECG changes may have resolved by the time the patient seeks medical assistance.

8. **B.** In a patient experiencing an ACS, inverted T waves suggest ischemia. T-wave inversion may precede the development of ST-segment changes, or they may occur simultaneously.

9. **A, C.** The term *extensive anterior MI* is used when an infarction involves the septum and anterior and lateral walls. ECG changes should be visible in leads V$_1$ through V$_6$, as well as leads I and aVL.

10. **D.** The term *high lateral infarction* is used to describe ST changes viewed in leads I and aVL. Reciprocal changes of a high lateral infarction can usually be seen in leads II, III, and aVF.

11. **A, F.** An inferior STEMI is present (as evidenced by the STE in leads II, III, and aVF); the ST-segment depression in leads I and aVL reflect reciprocal changes.

INTERPRETATION OF PRACTICE ECGs

Fig. 3.27

Rate and rhythm:	Sinus rhythm at 65 beats/min
STE:	II, III, aVF, V_3, V_4, V_5, V_6
ST depression:	I, aVL
Axis:	Normal
Interpretation:	Suspected inferolateral STEMI. Obtain V_4R to assess for RVI. Artifact in I and III.

Fig. 3.28

Rate and rhythm:	Sinus arrhythmia at 75 beats/min
Axis:	Normal
Interpretation:	Normal ECG. Artifact in I, II, III, aVL, aVF, and V_3.

Fig. 3.29

Rate and rhythm:	Sinus bradycardia at 59 beats/min
STE:	I, aVL, V_2 through V_6
T-wave changes:	Tall in V_2, V_3, V_4, V_5
Axis:	Normal
Interpretation:	Suspected anterolateral STEMI. Baseline wander in II and III.

Fig. 3.30

Rate and rhythm:	Sinus rhythm at 75 beats/min with occasional premature ventricular complexes (PVCs)
ST depression:	I, II, aVF, V_5, V_6
Axis:	Normal
Interpretation:	No evidence of STEMI. Artifact in III.

Fig. 3.31

Rate and rhythm:	Sinus rhythm at 90 beats/min
STE:	V_1 through V_4; borderline in III and aVF
T-wave changes:	Inverted in aVL
Pathologic Q waves:	V_1 through V_3
Axis:	Left
Interpretation:	Possible inferior, anteroseptal STEMI. STE in V_1 through V_4. Borderline STE in III and aVF. Poor R-wave progression. Left axis deviation. Artifact in aVR, aVL, and V_1. Obtain V_4R to assess for RVI.

Fig. 3.32

Rate and rhythm:	Sinus rhythm at 73 beats/min with occasional PVCs
STE:	V_2, V_3, V_4, V_5, V_6
ST depression:	III
T-wave changes:	Tall, peaked in V_2, V_3, V_4
Axis:	Normal
Interpretation:	Suspected anterior STEMI.

Fig. 3.33

Rate and rhythm:	Unable to determine
Interpretation:	Data quality prohibits interpretation; artifact in I, II, III, aVL, aVF, and V_1 through V_6.

Fig. 3.34

Rate and rhythm:	Sinus rhythm at 92 beats/min with occasional supraventricular premature complexes
STE:	V_2 through V_4; borderline in V_1 and V_5
ST depression:	II, III, aVF
Pathologic Q waves:	V_1, V_2
Axis:	Normal
Interpretation:	Suspected anteroseptal STEMI. Artifact in I, III, aVL, and aVF.

Fig. 3.35

Rate and rhythm:	89 beats/min
Interpretation:	Arm leads reversed (negative PQRST waveforms in I, positive PQRST waveforms in aVR). No further interpretation is possible.

INTERPRETATION OF CASE STUDIES

CASE STUDY 3.1

Although this patient is not complaining of chest pain or discomfort, she is presenting with anginal equivalent symptoms (e.g., sudden onset of shortness of breath, fatigue). Because chest pain or discomfort can develop at any time, be sure to ask her if these symptoms are present when obtaining repeat vital signs, and ask her to notify you if they occur.

The patient's 12-lead ECG shows evidence of an inferior STEMI (STE in leads II, III, and aVF and reciprocal ST depression in I and aVL). You should obtain a right-sided 12-lead ECG and determine if an RVI is present. Because borderline STE is present in leads V_3 through V_6, closely evaluate subsequent 12-lead ECGs for the development of a lateral infarction. Be alert for the development of complications of inferior infarction, such as bradydysrhythmias and AV blocks.

Obtain a portable chest radiograph and draw initial laboratory tests, including cardiac biomarkers, electrolytes, and coagulation studies. Because of the urgency for reperfusion in patients with STEMI, do not wait for biomarker results to begin treatment; use your clinical assessment and 12-lead ECG findings to determine initial treatment strategies. Use current STEMI treatment guidelines and algorithms to guide your management decisions, including pharmacologic reperfusion (i.e., fibrinolytics) or mechanical reperfusion (i.e., PCI) and medical therapies. Minimize the time to reperfusion by working quickly and efficiently. Repeat the 12-lead ECG when clinically indicated.

CASE STUDY 3.2

If there are no contraindications, give aspirin as soon as possible. An anteroseptal STEMI is suspected based on this patient's 12-lead ECG (i.e., STE observed in V_1 through V_5). Select a reperfusion strategy, obtain a portable chest radiograph, and draw initial laboratory studies.

Relief of the patient's chest pain is a priority. Recall that up to three doses of sublingual or aerosol NTG can be given at 3- to 5-minute intervals for patients with ischemic chest discomfort until the discomfort is relieved or the presence of hypotension limits its use. Closely monitor the patient's vital signs and ECG after each dose. Morphine may be needed to alleviate ischemic chest discomfort unresponsive to nitrates.

Six minutes after administering a sublingual NTG tablet to this patient, he rated his chest pain 9/10. Within 2 minutes of giving a second tablet, he rated his pain 6/10 and said, "I feel funny." Reassessment revealed a blood pressure of 90/60 mm Hg, a heart rate of 92 beats/min, and pale, clammy skin. After placing the patient supine and administering 200 mL of normal saline, his blood pressure was 120/74 mm Hg, his heart rate was 78 beats/min, and his skin was pink, warm, and dry. However, his chest pain increased to 10/10. He was taken to the cardiac catheterization laboratory for immediate PCI.

ST-Elevation Variants

aVR   V₁   V₄

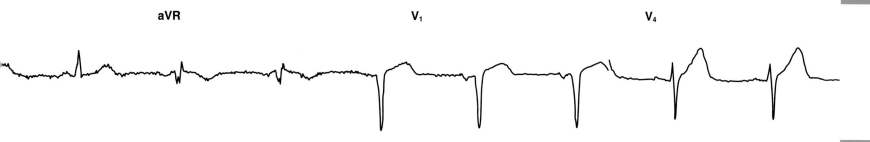

LEARNING OBJECTIVES

After reading this chapter, you should be able to:

1. Recognize that many conditions other than infarction may produce ST-segment elevation (STE).
2. Identify the electrocardiographic (ECG) criteria for left ventricular hypertrophy (LVH), bundle branch block (BBB), ventricular rhythms, early repolarization (ER), and pericarditis.
3. Recognize how the ST segment is displaced by LVH, left bundle branch block (LBBB), and ventricular rhythms.
4. Review the anatomy of the intraventricular conduction system.
5. Develop an approach to differentiating right bundle branch block (RBBB) from LBBB.
6. Describe the clinical presentation of pericarditis.

KEY TERMS

bundle branch block: A disruption in impulse conduction from the bundle of His through either the right or left bundle branch to the Purkinje fibers

cardiac enlargement: Situations in which one or more of the heart's chambers become bigger because of an increase in cavity volume, wall thickness, or both

terminal force: The final portion of the QRS complex

INTRODUCTION

Thus far, most examples of STE provided in this text have resulted from myocardial infarction (MI). This strategy was used to encourage your familiarity with the pattern(s) of MI. However, gross overdiagnosis would result if every instance of STE were interpreted as MI. MI produces STE because the infarction affects ventricular repolarization, ventricular depolarization, or both. Likewise, any condition that affects ventricular repolarization and/or depolarization can also produce STE. This chapter focuses on the following five conditions that can produce STE: LVH, BBB, ventricular rhythms (including paced ventricular rhythms), ER, and pericarditis (Fig. 4.1).

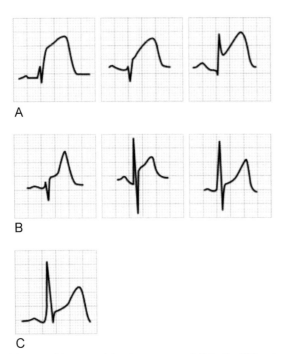

A

B

C

Fig. 4.1 Analysis of ST segment–T wave morphology in acute myocardial infarction (AMI), early repolarization (ER), and acute pericarditis. An analysis of the ST segment–T wave morphology (from the beginning at the J point to the end at the apex of the T wave) may be particularly helpful in distinguishing among the various causes of ST-segment elevation (STE) and identifying the STE cause. (A) The initial upsloping portion of the ST segment is usually either flat (horizontally or obliquely) or convex in the patient with ST-elevation myocardial infarction (STEMI). This morphologic observation, however, should be used only as a guideline; it is not infallible. (B) Non-AMI causes of STE are seen here with concavity of the ST segment–T wave (left ER, middle pericarditis, right ER). (C) Patients with STEMI may demonstrate concavity of this portion of the waveform. Serial ECGs may help determine if the presence of STE is pathologic. (From Walls, R. M., Hockberger, R. S., Gausche-Hill, M., Erickson, T. B., & Wilcox, S. R. [2023]. *Rosen's emergency medicine: Concepts and clinical practice.* [10th ed.]. Elsevier.)

VENTRICULAR HYPERTROPHY

Cardiac enlargement refers to situations in which one or more of the heart's chambers become bigger because of an increase in its cavity volume, wall thickness, or both (Goldberger et al., 2024). When enlargement occurs, the number of heart muscle fibers does not increase; instead the individual muscle fibers become larger (i.e., hypertrophied) (Goldberger et al., 2024). Hypertrophy is commonly accompanied by dilation. With dilation, the heart muscle cells typically become longer (Goldberger et al., 2024). Dilation may be acute or chronic. When evaluating the ECG for the presence of chamber enlargement, it is essential to check the calibration marker to ensure that it is 10 mm (1 mV) tall.

Right Ventricular Hypertrophy

With right ventricular hypertrophy (RVH), current travels between hypertrophied cells and moves through the enlarged right ventricle, producing higher-than-normal voltages on the body surface (Mirvis & Goldberger, 2022) (Fig. 4.2). Because the right ventricle is typically smaller than the left, it must become significantly enlarged before changes are visible on the ECG.

Several criteria have been proposed for detecting RVH on the ECG. Most involve assessing the height of the R waves in leads V_1 and V_2 and the depth of the S waves in V_5 and V_6 (Box 4.1, Fig. 4.3). RVH is often accompanied by right axis deviation and evidence of right atrial abnormality may be seen. In the limb and right chest leads, right atrial abnormality produces P waves that are tall (at least 2.5 mm), peaked, and usually of normal duration. RVH can mimic a posterior infarction on the ECG. Causes of RVH include pulmonary hypertension, chronic pulmonary diseases, pulmonary embolism, valvular heart disease, and congenital heart disease (e.g., atrial and ventricular septal defects).

Consider This

A *strain pattern*, defined as downsloping as ST-segment depression and T-wave inversion, may be observed on the ECGs of patients with chronic RVH or LVH. The strain pattern represents ventricular repolarization abnormalities. Right ventricular strain is usually observed in the inferior leads (i.e., II, III, aVF) and V_1 to V_4. Left ventricular strain is typically seen in leads I, aVL, and V_4 to V_6. Recognizing the presence of a right ventricular strain pattern is of value in patients with conditions such as pulmonary hypertension, pulmonary embolism, heart failure, and congenital heart disease. In addition, the presence of a left ventricular strain pattern has been used to identify patients at increased risk of cardiovascular complications, including MI, heart failure, ventricular dysrhythmias, and sudden death.

QRS in hypertrophy

V₁	V₆

Main QRS vector

Normal

LVH

RVH   or   or

Fig. **4.2** Left ventricular hypertrophy (LVH) increases the amplitude of electrical forces directed to the left and posteriorly. In addition, repolarization abnormalities can cause ST-segment depression and T-wave inversion in leads with a prominent R wave. Right ventricular hypertrophy (RVH) can shift the QRS vector to the right, usually with an RS, R, or qR complex in lead V₁, especially when caused by severe pressure overload. (From Libby, P., Bonow, R. O., Mann, D. L., Tomaselli, G. F., Bhatt, D. L., & Solomon, S. D. [2022]. *Braunwald's heart disease: A textbook of cardiovascular medicine* [12th ed.]. Elsevier.)

Box **4.1**	Examples of ECG Criteria for Right Ventricular Hypertrophy Recognition

- Tall R waves (7 mm or more) in V₁
- qR pattern in V₁
- Deeper-than-normal S waves (7 mm or more) in leads V₅ or V₆
- Right axis deviation usually present

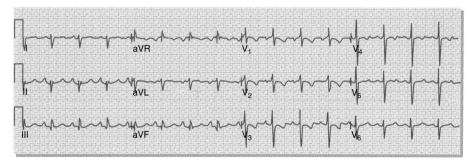

Fig. **4.3** Right ventricular hypertrophy with tall R wave in the right chest leads, downsloping ST depression in the chest leads, right axis deviation, and evidence of right atrial enlargement. (From Wing, E. J., & Schiffman, F. J. [2022]. *Cecil's essentials of medicine* [10th ed.]. Elsevier.)

Left Ventricular Hypertrophy

LVH is primarily recognized on the ECG by increased QRS amplitude accompanied by changes in the ST segment and T wave (see Fig. 4.2). Typically, R waves in leads facing the left ventricle (i.e., I, aVL, V₅, and V₆) are taller than normal, and S waves in leads V₁ and V₂ are deeper than normal (Mirvis & Goldberger, 2022). In addition, the QRS duration is often increased in LVH and may be attributed to the longer time required to activate the thickened wall of the left ventricle (Hancock et al., 2009) and the slower-than-normal conduction within the working myocardium. LVH may be accompanied by left axis deviation, prolongation of the QT interval, and evidence of left atrial abnormality. With left atrial abnormality, the middle and end of the P wave are prolonged, and notched P waves are usually visible (most easily seen in the limb leads). Common causes of LVH include hypertension, aortic stenosis or insufficiency, mitral insufficiency, and hypertrophic cardiomyopathy.

Several formulas exist to assist in LVH recognition. Recent studies have shown that adding the deepest S-wave amplitude in any lead and the S-wave amplitude in V₄ provides improved sensitivity and adequate specificity for the diagnosis of LVH compared with other criteria (Box 4.2). An example of LVH is shown in Fig. 4.4.

Box **4.2**	Examples of ECG Criteria for Left Ventricular Hypertrophy Recognition

- R wave in lead aVL is 11 mm or more
- R wave in lead aVF is 20 mm or more
- R wave in lead I + S wave in III is 25 mm or more
- S wave in lead III is 20 mm or more
- S wave in lead V₁ or V₂ is 30 mm or more
- S wave in V₁ + height of the tallest R wave in V₅ or V₆ is 35 mm or more
- S wave in lead V₂ + R wave in lead aVL is 20 mm or more in women, 28 mm or more in men
- S-wave amplitude in V₄ + deepest S wave in any lead is 23 mm or more in women, 28 mm or more in men

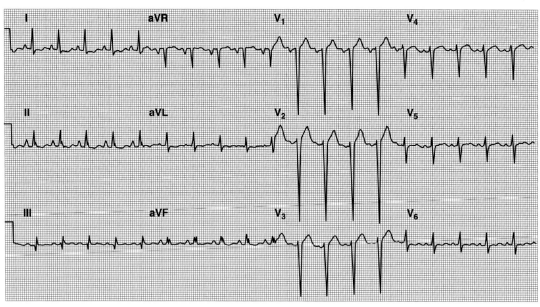

Fig. **4.4** Left ventricular hypertrophy. Note the ST-segment elevation in leads V_1, V_2, and V_3.

Note the STE in leads V_1, V_2, and V_3 and the ST-segment depression in leads V_5 and V_6. These ECG findings conform to a pattern shared by LVH, LBBB, and ventricular rhythms in which the QRS complex and the T wave are oppositely directed. In other words, the T wave points up when the QRS complex points down and vice versa. This phenomenon would hardly be noteworthy in a discussion of infarction except for one crucial fact: the T wave often "drags" the ST segment along with it. Thus when the QRS complex is primarily negative, the T wave will be positively deflected, and it can drag the ST segment up with it. This is how LVH, LBBB, and ventricular rhythms can masquerade as an infarction. Additionally, the negative deflection may produce a Q wave or QS complex equal to 40 milliseconds (msec) or more in duration. This further clouds the interpretation by giving the appearance of pathologic Q waves. Therefore, careful correlation of the patient's ECG, clinical presentation, and the results of other diagnostic studies are essential.

A 12-lead ECG's interpretive algorithm checks for the presence of LVH using preprogrammed criteria, including formulas, to measure voltage. If the 12-lead machine determines that an ECG meets the criteria for LVH, a message is displayed, such as "Meets voltage criteria for left ventricular hypertrophy." In contrast, a message such as "Possible criteria for left ventricular hypertrophy with repolarization abnormality" does *not* mean the same thing.

Consider This

When applying the criteria for LVH based on QRS amplitude, keep in mind that several factors other than the size or mass of the left ventricle can influence QRS voltages. These factors include age, sex, race, body habitus (i.e., obesity), and the sites of ECG electrode placement (Hancock et al., 2009).

BUNDLE BRANCH BLOCKS

Structures of the Intraventricular Conduction System

After passing through the atrioventricular (AV) node, the electrical impulse enters the bundle of His, which is normally the only electrical connection between the atria and the ventricles. It is located in the upper portion of the interventricular septum and connects the AV node with the two bundle branches (Fig. 4.5). A **BBB** is a disruption in impulse conduction from the bundle of His through either the right or left bundle branch to the Purkinje fibers. A BBB may be intermittent or permanent, complete or incomplete.

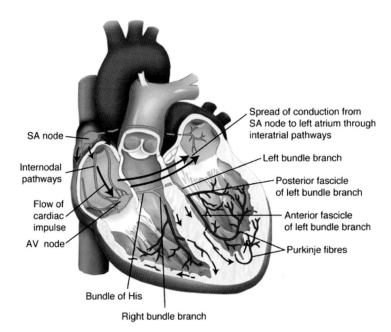

Fig. **4.5** Cardiac conduction system. *AV,* Atrioventricular; *SA,* sinoatrial. (From Lewis, S. L., Bucher, L., Heitkemper, M. M., Harding, M. M., Kwong, J., & Roberts, D. [2017]. *Medical-surgical nursing: Assessment and management of clinical problems.* [10th ed.]. Elsevier.)

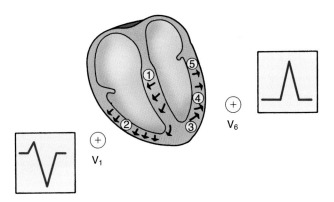

Fig. **4.6** Sequence of normal ventricular depolarization and resulting QRS complex, as seen in leads V₁ and V₆. (From Urden, L. D., Stacy, K. M., & Lough, M. E. [2022]. *Critical care nursing: Diagnosis and management* [9th ed.]. Elsevier.)

The right bundle branch travels down the right side of the interventricular septum to conduct the electrical impulse to the right ventricle. Structurally, the right bundle branch is long, thin, and more fragile than the left. Because of its structure, a relatively small lesion in the right bundle branch can result in delays or interruptions in electrical impulse transmission.

The left bundle branch begins as a short and thick bundle of nervous tissue and then divides into two subdivisions, the anterior and posterior fascicles. The fascicles branch into networks of Purkinje fibers. The anterior fascicle receives its blood supply from septal branches of the left anterior descending (LAD) artery. It spreads the electrical impulse to the anterior and lateral portions of the left ventricle. This fascicle is thin and vulnerable to disruptions in electrical impulse transmission. In contrast, impulse transmission in the posterior fascicle is rarely disrupted because it is short, thick, and receives a dual blood supply from the LAD and the right coronary artery. This fascicle relays the impulse to the inferior and posterior portions of the left ventricle.

Bundle Branch Activation

The wave of normal ventricular depolarization moves from the endocardium to the epicardium. The left side of the interventricular septum, which is stimulated by the left posterior fascicle, is stimulated first. The electrical impulse (i.e., wave of depolarization) then traverses the septum to stimulate the right side. The left and right ventricles are then depolarized simultaneously (Fig. 4.6).

A delay or block can occur in any part of the intraventricular conduction system. If a delay or block occurs in one of the bundle branches, the ventricles do not depolarize at the same time. Instead, the electrical impulse travels first down the unblocked branch and stimulates that ventricle. Because of the block, the impulse must then travel from cell to cell through the myocardium, rather than through the normal conduction pathway, to stimulate the other ventricle. The ventricle with the blocked bundle branch is the last to be depolarized.

Significance of Bundle Branch Block

Because the LAD artery supplies much of the bundle branches, patients experiencing septal and anteroseptal infarctions are most likely to develop BBB. Of course, a patient experiencing an acute coronary syndrome (ACS) and presenting with BBB may have had the BBB as a preexisting condition. Unless a previous ECG is available for comparison or the BBB develops during the ACS, it can be challenging to determine which came first, the ACS or the BBB. When an infarction causes BBB, it can progress to a complete AV block with a slow ventricular rate. LBBB is significant because of its ability to produce STE and wide Q waves that resemble infarction, thereby complicating the ECG recognition of acute MI.

Electrocardiographic Criteria

When one of the bundles becomes blocked, the impulse normally conducted by that bundle branch is interrupted and does not depolarize the intended ventricle. Meanwhile, the other bundle branch is conducting its impulse and depolarizing its respective ventricle. How does the other ventricle depolarize? Very slowly. For the second ventricle to depolarize, the electrical impulses must trudge through myocardial cells, which are not specialized for electrical conduction. Thus the impulses from one ventricle must be transmitted, cell by cell, to the other. As a result, ventricular depolarization takes longer because the impulses are wading through the muck and mire and not traveling down the normal conduction pathway. This delay is evidenced in the form of a wide QRS complex.

Consider This

Whereas BBB increases the *width* of the QRS complex, LVH increases the *amplitude* because of the increase in electrical activity due to the thicker ventricle.

Essentially, two conditions must exist to suspect BBB (Box 4.3). First, the QRS complex must have an abnormal duration (i.e., 120 msec or more in duration if a complete BBB); second, the QRS complex must arise as the result of supraventricular activity (this excludes paced beats and beats that originate from the ventricles). If these two conditions are met, delayed ventricular conduction is assumed to be present, and BBB is the most common (but not the only) cause of this abnormal conduction.

Variation in QRS duration from lead to lead is often seen and may produce confusion about whether the complex is or is not wide. Some complexes appear narrow in some leads but, when measured, are just as wide as the other leads. Therefore, *measure the QRS complex duration. Do not trust only your eyes.* Try to pinpoint the exact beginning and end of the QRS complex, although this can be difficult and is sometimes impossible. Therefore, *when measuring for BBB, select the widest QRS complex with a discernible beginning and end.*

The criteria for BBB recognition may be found in any lead of the ECG. However, when differentiating RBBB from LBBB, consider the QRS morphology (i.e., shape) in specific leads. For example, lead V_1 is probably the best lead to use when differentiating between RBBB and LBBB.

Box 4.3   ECG Criteria for Bundle Branch Block Recognition

To be considered a BBB, the following ECG criteria must be met:
- QRS duration of 120 msec or more in adults (if a *complete* RBBB or LBBB); if a BBB pattern is discernible and the QRS duration is between 110 and 119 msec in adults, it is called an *incomplete* right or left BBB (Kusumoto et al., 2019). (If the QRS is wide but there is no BBB pattern, the term *wide QRS* or *intraventricular conduction delay* is used to describe the QRS.)
- Visible QRS complexes are produced by supraventricular activity (i.e., the QRS complex is not a paced beat and does not originate in the ventricles).

Differentiating RBBB From LBBB

Once BBB is suspected, examining V_1 can reveal whether the block affects the right or left bundle branch. Following are descriptions of how each type of block affects the direction of electrical current and produces its own distinct QRS morphology.

Right Bundle Branch Block

In RBBB, the electrical impulse travels through the AV node and down the left bundle branch into the interventricular septum. The left posterior fascicle activates the septum and depolarizes in a left-to-right direction (i.e., toward V_1), producing an initial small R wave (Fig. 4.7). As the left bundle continues to conduct impulses, the entire left ventricle is depolarized from right to left, producing movement away from V_1, and resulting in a negative deflection (i.e., an S wave). The impulses that depolarize the left ventricle conduct through the myocardial cells and then depolarize the right ventricle, creating a movement of electrical activity in the direction of V_1, so a second positive deflection is recorded (R′). The resulting small r, deep S, tall R (rSR′) pattern is characteristic of RBBB. The rSR′ pattern, sometimes called an "M" or "rabbit ear" pattern, is characteristic of RBBB (Fig. 4.8), although other pattern variations are possible. To summarize, the ECG characteristics of RBBB include the following (Kusumoto et al., 2019):

- rsr′, rsR′, rSR′, or (rarely) a small q, tall R (qR) pattern in leads V_1 or V_2
- S wave of greater duration than the R wave or more than 40 msec in leads I and V_6
- QRS duration of 120 msec or more if a complete RBBB; a QRS duration between 110 and 119 msec if incomplete

Although RBBB can occur in individuals with no underlying heart disease, acute RBBB may occur secondary to an acute anteroseptal infarction, heart failure, pericarditis, myocarditis, or pulmonary embolism. Chronic RBBB may be caused by coronary artery disease.

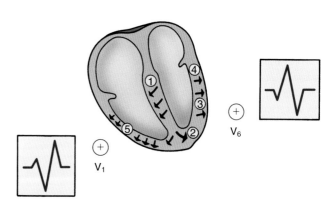

Fig. **4.7** Sequence of ventricular depolarization for a right bundle branch block and resulting QRS complex, as seen in leads V_1 and V_6. (From Urden, L. D., Stacy, K. M., & Lough, M. E. [2022]. *Critical care nursing: Diagnosis and management* [9th ed.]. Elsevier.)

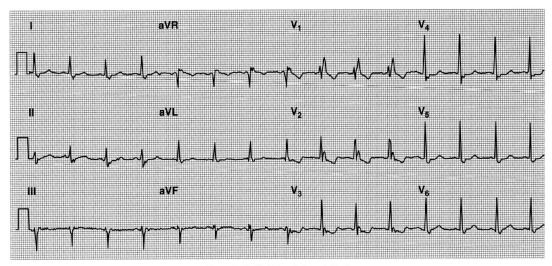

Fig. **4.8** Right bundle branch block.

disease, cardiac surgery, degenerative disease of the heart's conduction system, or congenital cardiac disorders, such as atrial and ventricular septal defects.

Left Bundle Branch Block

In LBBB, the right bundle branch depolarizes the septum and right ventricle. The septum is part of the left ventricle and is normally depolarized by the left bundle branch. Because the left bundle branch is blocked, depolarization of the septum by the right bundle branch occurs in an abnormal direction (i.e., from right to left); thus the wave of myocardial depolarization begins with the net movement of current going away from V_1 and is recorded as an initial negative deflection (Fig. 4.9). The right ventricle is depolarized next. Because the wave of depolarization moves briefly toward the positive electrode in lead V_1, a small upright notch in the QRS complex is seen on the ECG. As the remainder of the left ventricle is depolarized, the QRS complex is inscribed in lead V_1 as a deep negative deflection (i.e., an S wave), reflecting the left ventricle's large muscle mass. Sometimes, depolarization of the left ventricle overshadows the right ventricle on the ECG. When this occurs, a QS deflection is inscribed in lead V_1, and the small upright notch that is usually seen with right ventricular depolarization is absent (Fig. 4.10). Unfortunately, not every BBB presents with a clear RSR′ or QS pattern in V_1. Often the pattern more closely resembles a qR pattern or an rS pattern (Fig. 4.11), making the differentiation less clear.

The ECG characteristics of complete LBBB include the following (Kusumoto et al., 2019):

- QRS duration of 120 msec or more
- Broad notched or slurred R wave in leads I, aVL, V_5, and V_6 and an occasional RS (tall R, deep S) pattern in V_5 and V_6

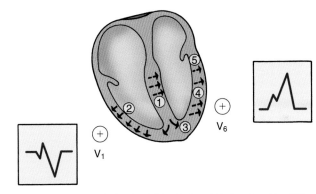

Fig. **4.9** Sequence of ventricular depolarization for a left bundle branch block and resulting QRS complex, as seen in leads V_1 and V_6. (From Urden, L. D., Stacy, K. M., & Lough, M. E. [2022]. *Critical care nursing: Diagnosis and management* [9th ed.]. Elsevier.)

- Absent Q waves in leads I, V_5, and V_6, but a narrow Q wave may be present in the absence of myocardial pathology in lead aVL
- ST depression in leads I, aVL, V_5, and V_6; STE in leads V_1 to V_3
- Inverted T waves in leads I, aVL, V_5, and V_6; positive T waves in V_1 to V_3; T waves are usually opposite in direction to QRS (i.e., discordant)

The ECG characteristics of incomplete LBBB include the following (Kusumoto et al., 2019):

- QRS duration between 110 and 119 msec
- Presence of LVH pattern
- Absent Q waves in leads I, V_5, and V_6

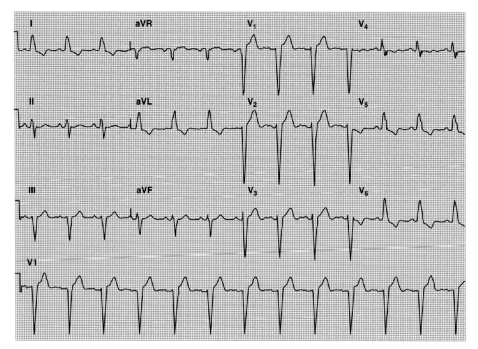

Fig. **4.10** Left bundle branch block.

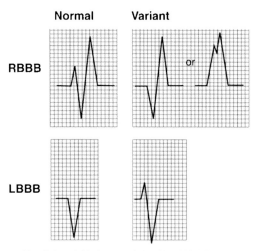

Fig. **4.11** Variant patterns of bundle branch block as seen in lead V$_1$. *LBBB*, Left bundle branch block; *RBBB*, right bundle branch block.

LBBB may be acute or chronic. Acute LBBB may occur secondary to anteroseptal MI, acute heart failure, acute pericarditis or myocarditis, or acute cardiac trauma. Chronic LBBB may occur because of hypertensive heart disease, severe coronary artery disease, and aortic stenosis. Nonischemic diseases, such as Lev's disease and Lenègre's disease, can also produce a BBB. Lev's disease produces BBB by calcifying the heart's fibrous skeleton. The fibrous skeleton is the infrastructure to which the muscles and valves are attached. Portions of the conduction system are located near the fibrous skeleton or may pass through it. If the fibrous skeleton begins to calcify, part of the electrical conduction system may become "pinched," resulting in a block. Lenègre's disease is a more diffuse sclerodegenerative disease that tends to affect the distal portions of the conduction system but may also affect the more proximal portions. This process occurs with age, is unrelated to ischemic heart disease, and is sometimes called the "graying" of the electrical conduction system.

An Easier Way

Remember that in the setting of BBB, the ventricles are not depolarized in their usual simultaneous manner. Instead, they are depolarized sequentially. The last ventricle to be depolarized is, of course, the ventricle with the blocked bundle branch. Therefore, if it is possible to determine the ventricle that was depolarized last, it becomes possible to determine the bundle branch that was blocked. For example, if the right ventricle was depolarized last, it is because the impulse traveled down the left bundle branch, depolarized the left ventricle first, then marched through and depolarized the right ventricle.

It stands to reason that if one ventricle is depolarized late, its depolarization makes up the latter part of the QRS complex. The final portion of the QRS complex is called the **terminal force**. Examination of the terminal force of the QRS complex reveals the ventricle that was depolarized last and, therefore, the blocked bundle branch.

To identify the terminal force, first locate the J point. Then, from the J point, move backward into the QRS and determine if the last electrical activity produced an upward or downward deflection. An example of the terminal force in both RBBB and LBBB is illustrated in Fig. 4.12. If the right bundle branch is blocked, the right ventricle will be depolarized last, and the current will move from the left ventricle to the right, creating a positive deflection in the terminal force of the QRS complex in V$_1$. On the other hand, if the left bundle branch is blocked, the left ventricle will be depolarized last, and the current will flow from right to left, producing a negative deflection in the terminal force of the QRS complex seen in V$_1$. Therefore, to differentiate RBBB from LBBB, look at V$_1$ and determine whether the terminal force of the QRS complex is directed upward or downward. If it is directed upward, RBBB is present (i.e., the current is moving toward the right ventricle and toward V$_1$). On the other hand, LBBB is present when the terminal force of the QRS complex is directed downward (i.e., the current is moving away from V$_1$ and toward the left ventricle). This rule is beneficial when RSR′ and QS variants are present.

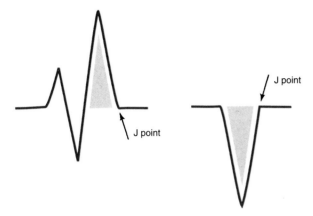

Fig. **4.12** Determining the direction of the terminal force. In lead V₁, move from the J point into the QRS complex and determine whether the terminal portion (last 0.04 second) of the QRS complex is a positive (upright) or negative (downward) deflection. If the two criteria for bundle branch block are met, and the terminal portion of the QRS is positive, a right bundle branch block is most likely present. If the terminal portion of the QRS is negative, a left bundle branch block is most likely present.

A simple way to remember this rule has been suggested by Mike Taigman and Syd Canan and is demonstrated in Fig. 4.13. They recognized the similarity between this rule and the turn indicator on a car. When a right turn is made, the turn indicator is lifted. Likewise, when an RBBB is present, the terminal force of the QRS complex points up. Conversely, left turns and LBBB are directed downward.

Concordance

When analyzing a BBB, *concordance* refers to ST segments and T waves that deflect in the same direction as the terminal (last) portion of the QRS complex. Normally, a BBB produces *discordant* ST segments and T waves. In other words, the ST segments and T waves are in the opposite direction of the terminal portion of the QRS complex. Concordant STE is almost always abnormal with a BBB.

Sgarbossa Criteria

In 1996, Dr. Elena Sgarbossa and colleagues published a study that tested ECG criteria for diagnosing acute MI in the presence of LBBB (Sgarbossa et al., 1996). These ECG criteria include the following:
1. STE of 1 mm or more that is concordant with (i.e., in the same direction as) the QRS complex in any lead (5 points)
2. Concordant ST-segment depression of 1 mm or more in lead V₁, V₂, and/or V₃ (3 points)
3. STE of 5 mm or more that is discordant with (i.e., in the opposite direction from) a negative QRS complex in any lead (2 points)

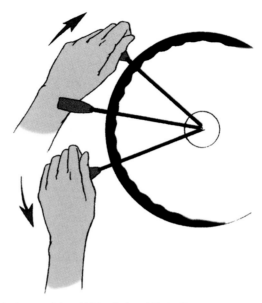

Fig. **4.13** Differentiating between right and left bundle branch blocks. The "turn signal" theory is that right is up and left is down.

To improve diagnostic accuracy, the Sgarbossa criteria have been modified; specifically, the 5-mm discordant STE requirement has been replaced with a proportion. The Smith-modified Sgarbossa criteria include the following (Smith et al., 2012):
1. One or more leads with a positive QRS complex and concordant STE of 1 mm or more
2. Concordant ST-segment depression of 1 mm or more in lead V₁, V₂, and/or V₃
3. One or more leads with 1 mm or more STE and proportionally excessive discordant STE (STE of at least 25% or more of the depth of the preceding S wave)

The modified Sgarbossa criteria do not use a point system; if any modified ECG criteria are met, the result is considered positive, and the cardiac catheterization laboratory should be activated.

Exceptions

Two notable exceptions must be mentioned to complete the discussion of BBB. The first involves the criteria used to recognize BBB, whereas the second relates to differentiating LBBB from RBBB.

The criteria used to recognize BBB are valid but lack some sensitivity and specificity. Junctional rhythms can limit sensitivity because there may be no discernible P waves when the AV junction is the pacemaker site. The AV junction is a supraventricular pacemaker, but this presents as an exception to the two-part rule of BBB recognition. Specificity is limited by Wolff-Parkinson-White (WPW) syndrome and other conditions

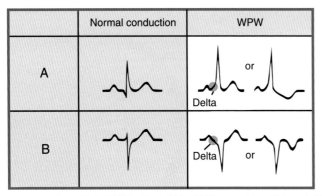

	Normal conduction	WPW
A		or
		Delta
B		Delta or

Fig. **4.14** Characteristic findings with the Wolff-Parkinson-White (WPW) pattern (short PR interval, QRS widening, and delta wave) compared with normal conduction. (A) The usual appearance of WPW in leads where the QRS complex is mainly upright. (B) The usual appearance of WPW when the QRS is predominantly negative. Negative delta waves may simulate pathologic Q waves, mimicking myocardial infarction. (From Grauer, K. [1998]. *A practical guide to ECG interpretation* [2nd ed.]. Mosby.)

that produce wide QRS complexes resulting from atrial activity. If the characteristic delta wave and shortened PR interval are recognized (Fig. 4.14), WPW syndrome should be suspected. However, this exception should not present too great a concern because the incidence of WPW syndrome is low. Similarly, hyperkalemia and other conditions that can widen the QRS are relatively infrequent.

As for differentiating LBBB from RBBB, a third category exists: nonspecific intraventricular conduction delay (NICD). In adults, NICD is described as a QRS duration of more than 110 msec, but the typical V_1 morphologies generally produced by RBBB or LBBB are absent (Kusumoto et al., 2019). NICD may occur due to an incomplete BBB, genetic predisposition, cardiomyopathies (ischemic or hypertensive) affecting the conduction system, or regional myocardial scarring caused by fibrosis, LVH, or a previous MI. Research shows that in individuals who are 30 years or older, LBBB and NICD are associated with a more than threefold risk of new-onset heart failure (Rankinen et al., 2020).

Consider This

The patient's clinical presentation is of little value in recognizing BBB because a ventricular conduction delay does not produce any clinical signs or symptoms. The underlying cause of a BBB may present with specific symptoms, but it does not help to identify the existence of a BBB. Therefore, rely on the ECG criteria to recognize the presence of BBB.

Fascicular Blocks

A block in only one of the fascicles of the bundle branches is called a *monofascicular block*. A block in any two divisions of the bundle branches is called a *bifascicular block*.

Although this term can describe a block in both the anterior and posterior branches of the left bundle branch, it is more commonly used to describe a combination of an RBBB and a left anterior fascicular block (LAFB) or a left posterior fascicular block (LPFB).

Left Anterior Fascicular Block

LAFB, also called *left anterior hemiblock*, is relatively common. With LAFB, the septum is depolarized in a left-to-right direction, which is normal. Impulse conduction usually occurs down the right bundle branch and into the right ventricle. Because conduction in the anterior fascicle of the left bundle branch is impaired, the posterior fascicle of the left ventricle is activated first. The electrical impulse then spreads in an upward and leftward direction to depolarize the anterior and lateral walls of the left ventricle. Despite the ventricular activation sequence change, the overall conduction time (i.e., the QRS duration) is usually less than 120 msec because only a portion of the left bundle branch is affected.

ECG characteristics of LAFB include the following (Kusumoto et al., 2019):
- Left axis deviation between −45 degree and −90 degree
- Small q, tall R (qR) pattern in lead aVL
- Small r, deep S (rS) pattern in leads II, III, and aVF
- QRS duration less than 120 msec

To quickly identify LAFB, look at leads I and aVF (Fig. 4.15). Left axis deviation is present if the QRS is positive in lead I and negative in aVF. Next, look at lead aVL for a qR pattern. This pattern may also be seen in lead I. An rS pattern may be seen in the inferior leads (i.e., II, III, and aVF). Finally, measure the QRS duration. With LAFB, the QRS duration is typically less than 120 msec.

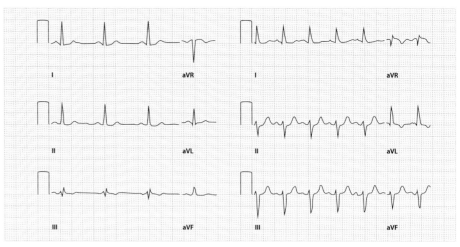

Fig. **4.15** Two electrocardiograms of a 50-year-old man recorded one day apart, before and after the development of left anterior fascicular block. (From Surawicz, B., & Knilans, T. K. [2008]. *Chou's electrocardiography in clinical practice* [6th ed.]. Saunders.)

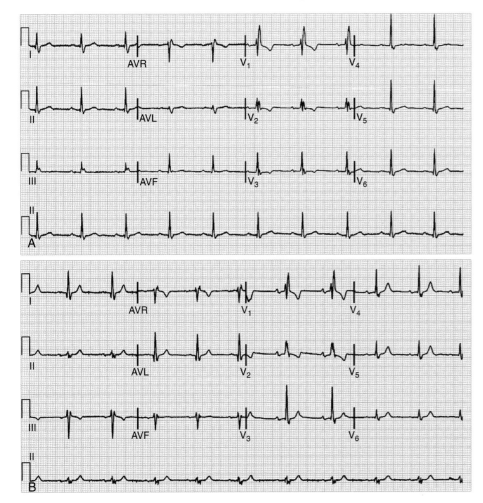

Fig. **4.16** Right bundle branch block (RBBB) versus bifascicular block. (A) A 12-lead ECG showing RBBB. Note an rsR′ pattern with the tall R′ in leads V₁ and V₂ and the broad S waves in leads I, V₅, and V₆. (B) Compare with this ECG showing bifascicular block. In addition to RBBB, note the left axis deviation and deep S waves in leads III and aVF, typical of left anterior fascicular block. (From Feather, A., Randall, D., & Waterhouse, M. [2021]. *Kumar and Clark's clinical medicine* [10th ed.]. Elsevier.)

LAFB is sometimes associated with RBBB (Fig. 4.16). In addition, LAFB may be seen in patients with aortic valve disease, coronary artery disease, hypertension, age-related degenerative disease of the bundle branch, and dilated cardiomyopathy.

Left Posterior Fascicular Block

LPFB, also called *left posterior hemiblock*, rarely occurs by itself. It more commonly occurs with RBBB (Fig. 4.17). With LPFB, impulse conduction occurs normally down

the right bundle branch and into the right ventricle. The anterior fascicle is activated first in the left ventricle, depolarizing the anterior and lateral walls. The impulse then spreads downward and rightward, resulting in right axis deviation. The posterior wall of the left ventricle and, ultimately, the interventricular septum are then depolarized. As with LAFB, the QRS duration is usually less than 120 msec because only a portion of the left bundle branch is affected.

ECG characteristics of LPFB include the following (Kusumoto et al., 2019):
- Right axis deviation between 90 degree and 180 degree
- Small r, deep S (rS) pattern in leads I and aVL
- Small q, tall R (qR) pattern in leads III and aVF
- QRS duration less than 120 msec

LPFB most often occurs in patients with coronary artery disease but can occur in patients with hypertension and valvular disease. Experts recommend that a diagnosis of LPFB be made only after other causes of right axis deviation have been ruled out, such as normal variants, mechanical shifts associated with inspiration or emphysema, RVH, chronic obstructive pulmonary disease, and acute or chronic pulmonary thromboembolism.

VENTRICULAR RHYTHMS

Impulses originating in the ventricles may result from either natural pacemaker sites or implanted pacemakers. Just as with BBB, ventricular rhythms may exhibit STE unrelated to infarct-related causes. This imitation STE is seen when the QRS complex is negatively deflected.

Ventricular-Paced Rhythm

In many ways, a ventricular-paced beat is a manmade LBBB. Consider that, when LBBB occurs, the electrical impulse travels down the right bundle branch and depolarizes the right ventricle, and the impulse spreads through the myocardium to depolarize the left ventricle. Pacemakers are usually introduced into the right ventricle and attached to the right ventricular wall. When the pacemaker fires, it sends its impulse into the right ventricle, which depolarizes, and the impulse is spread through the myocardium to depolarize the left ventricle. An example of a ventricular-paced rhythm-producing STE is shown in Fig. 4.18.

Similarly, spontaneous impulses originating in the ventricles can produce STE, which is often seen accompanying a negatively deflected premature ventricular complex. If a ventricular rhythm is present, the ECG may show STE in the leads that are negatively deflected.

The 12-lead ECG machine does an excellent job of measuring QRS width. A QRS of normal duration results when the ventricles contract simultaneously. A QRS of prolonged duration results when the ventricles contract sequentially. Both BBB and ventricular

Fig. **4.17** Bifascicular block (right bundle branch block [RBBB] with left posterior fascicular block). The chest leads show a typical RBBB pattern, while the limb leads show prominent right axis deviation (RAD). The combination of these two findings (in the absence of other more common causes of RAD, such as right ventricular hypertrophy or lateral myocardial infarction [MI]) is consistent with chronic bifascicular block due to left posterior fascicular block in concert with RBBB. This elderly patient had severe coronary artery disease. In addition, the prominent Q waves in leads III and aVF suggest underlying inferior wall MI. (From Goldberger, A. L., Goldberger, Z. D., & Shvilkin, A. [2024]. *Goldberger's clinical electrocardiography: A simplified approach* [10th ed.]. Elsevier.)

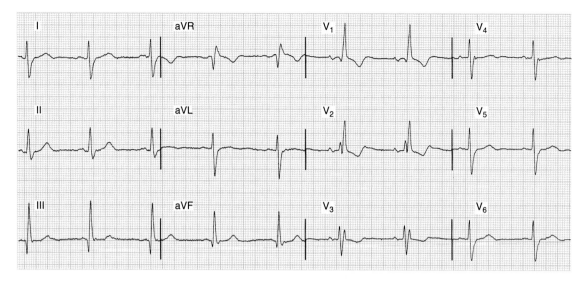

Fig. **4.18** Example of a ventricular-paced rhythm producing paced ST-segment elevation.

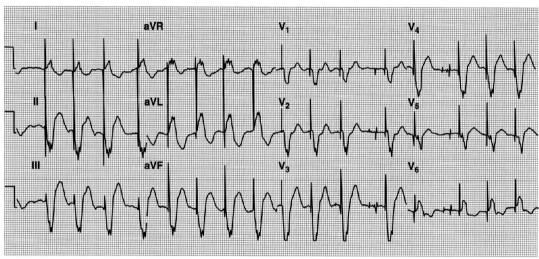

rhythms widen the QRS complex. If the QRS is of normal duration, no complete BBB or ventricular rhythm exists.

Consider This

Expect to see discordant ST segments and T waves (ST segments and T waves in the opposite direction of the last portion of the QRS complex) in ventricular rhythms and ventricular-paced rhythms because ventricular depolarization is abnormal.

EARLY REPOLARIZATION

ER is an ECG variant that closely resembles pericarditis or an anterior or anterolateral infarction on the ECGs of healthy, asymptomatic patients. Although ER is typically benign, there have been reports of its association with ventricular dysrhythmias and sudden cardiac arrest in some patients. In such cases, it is called early repolarization syndrome (ERS).

Electrocardiographic Criteria

Like the other conditions discussed in this chapter, ER can produce STE. Experts suggest that the ECG criteria shown in Box 4.4 be used when identifying an ER pattern (Antzelevitch et al., 2017). In healthy adults with ER, J-point elevation is usually followed by STE with a rapidly upsloping (ascending) shape and accompanied by a slur or notch at the end of the QRS just before and including the J point. Additionally, ER produces tall T waves resembling those seen in the hyperacute phase of MI (Fig. 4.19).

Clinical Presentation

ER is an ECG variant believed to be caused by increased vagal tone and is most prevalent in young, healthy individuals, especially African American men and athletes.

Box **4.4**	Typical ECG Characteristics of Early Repolarization

- Widespread STE with rapidly upsloping (ascending) shape of the initial portion of the ST segment that is typically maximal in leads V_2 to V_5
- Notching at the end of the QRS complex (J point) or slurring on the downstroke of the R wave
- Concordant T waves of large amplitude
- QRS duration less than 120 msec

Whereas ER is a common STE variant, ERS and Brugada syndrome (BrS) are repolarization abnormalities that predispose the patient to ventricular dysrhythmias (e.g., polymorphic ventricular tachycardia, ventricular fibrillation) and sudden cardiac arrest. ERS and BrS are inherited J-wave syndromes caused by mutations in one of several genes that predominantly affect males. With regard to ERS, horizontal/descending ST segments after the J point are associated with an increased risk of dysrhythmias (Rosso et al., 2012). Cardiac arrest may be the first symptom for patients with BrS or ERS (Antzelevitch et al., 2017). With both syndromes, cardiac arrest usually occurs during sleep or low levels of physical activity, with the highest incidence occurring in males between 30 and 50 years of age (Antzelevitch et al., 2017).

The Brugada pattern is characterized by coved (downsloping) or saddle-shaped STE of 2 mm or more and inverted T waves in more than one right chest lead (i.e., V_1 to V_3) (Fig. 4.20). This pattern of ECG changes is called BrS when it occurs in the presence of documented ventricular dysrhythmias, symptoms associated with dysrhythmias (e.g., syncope, seizures), or a family history of sudden cardiac death in family members younger than 45 years of age (Abbas et al., 2019).

Fig. **4.19** Early repolarization. Note the upwardly concave ST-segment elevation, best seen in leads V_4 to V_6. The T waves are relatively large in the same leads. Subtle notching is also seen at the J point in leads V_4 and V_5.

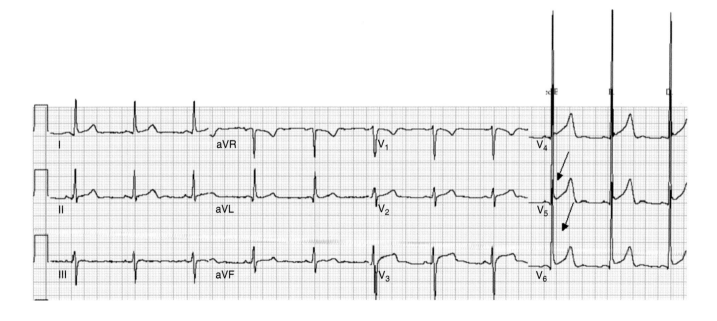

Brugada Pattern

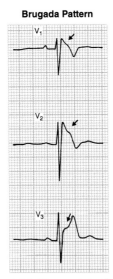

Fig. **4.20** Brugada pattern showing characteristic ST-segment elevation (STE) in leads V₁ to V₃. The ECG superficially resembles a right bundle branch block (RBBB) pattern. However, typical RBBB produces an rSR′ pattern in the right chest leads and is *not* associated with STE *(arrows)* in this distribution. The Brugada pattern appears to be a marker of abnormal right ventricular repolarization. Brugada syndrome is associated with an increased risk of life-threatening ventricular dysrhythmias and sudden cardiac arrest in some individuals. (From Goldberger, A. L., Goldberger, Z. D., & Shvilkin, A. [2024]. *Goldberger's clinical electrocardiography: A simplified approach* [10th ed.]. Elsevier.)

An implantable cardioverter-defibrillator is currently the mainstay of therapy to prevent sudden cardiac death for patients with ERS and BrS. In addition, quinidine, phosphodiesterase III inhibitors, and isoproterenol have been used to reduce the incidence of dysrhythmias in both syndromes.

PERICARDITIS

Another cause of STE is pericarditis. In this case, portions of the pericardium become inflamed, as does the adjoining epicardial surface of the heart. When STE occurs as the result of that inflammation, it is not the result of coronary artery disease. Anyone can develop pericarditis, but patients who are post-MI and post–cardiac surgery are especially susceptible.

Electrocardiographic Criteria

Pericarditis can produce several changes in the ECG. First, because the STE is related to scattered patches of inflammation around the pericardium and is not caused by an occluded coronary artery, STE is usually diffuse and not strictly grouped into anatomically contiguous leads.

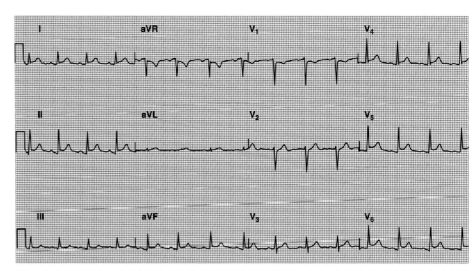

Fig. **4.21** The pattern of pericarditis. Note the diffuse pattern of ST-segment elevation, PR-segment depression in lead II, and J-point notching in leads II, V₅, and V₆.

Second, pericarditis can produce PR-segment depression. When the ST segment is compared with a depressed PR segment, it can give the appearance of STE. Using the TP segment to establish the isoelectric line will minimize this illusion. The presence of PR-segment elevation in lead aVR, with reciprocal PR-segment depression in other leads, is a crucial ECG clue in recognizing acute pericarditis (Mirvis & Goldberger, 2022).

Third, pericarditis can cause notching of the J point. Although not exclusive to pericarditis, J-point notching signifies the possibility of a noninfarct cause of STE. Fig. 4.21 illustrates how some leads show examples of true STE, whereas other leads appear elevated because of PR-segment depression, and a few display J-point notching.

Clinical Presentation

Chest pain is commonly the chief complaint in pericarditis. The pain is often described as "sharp" (the term *sharp* is intended to convey a knifelike pain, not to convey intensity) or "stabbing," unlike the more typical "pressure" or "heaviness" accompanying infarction. The pain of pericarditis can often be localized with one finger. In contrast, the discomfort associated with acute MI is typically over a larger area that cannot be localized with one finger. The pain of pericarditis tends to be affected by movement, ventilation, and position. The patient may state that the pain is minimized by leaning forward and intensified by lying supine. If pain radiation occurs, the patient may report that it is felt about the base of the neck or the area between the shoulder blades.

TABLE 4.1	Clinical Presentation of Acute Myocardial Infarction and Pericarditis	
Finding	**Myocardial Infarction**	**Pericarditis**
Chest pain (nature)	Pressure	Sharp, stabbing
Chest pain (radiation)	Left arm, shoulder, jaw	Base of neck, trapezius area
Chest pain (aggravation)	Unaffected by movement	Affected by movement, ventilation, swallowing, etc.; may improve when leaning forward
STE	Appears in anatomically contiguous leads	Diffuse across ECG, may occur in leads not grouped anatomically
PR-segment depression	Uncommon	Common, may give appearance of STE

ECG, Electrocardiogram.

The recognizable ECG features of pericarditis are subtle and can easily be overlooked or misinterpreted. Therefore, it is often the clinical presentation of pericarditis that is first recognized. Once pericarditis is suspected, the ECG can be closely examined (or reexamined) for substantiating evidence. Table 4.1 compares the ECG and clinical features of MI and pericarditis.

Although ER and pericarditis can cause STE, neither condition is particularly good at causing reciprocal changes. If STE is present on the ECG and clear, obvious reciprocal changes are present, it is reasonable to scratch ER and pericarditis from the list of possible causes of STE.

WHAT SHOULD YOU DO NOW?

It is sometimes challenging to differentiate between infarct and noninfarct causes of STE. In addition, some cases can be decided only after hours of observation, serial ECGs, and extensive testing. Therefore, don't expect that a single ECG will always provide enough information to determine the cause of STE.

Remember that the ECG simply records the electrical current on the patient's skin. For this reason, the ECG is not always sensitive enough to detect subtle changes and is not always specific enough to differentiate between certain conditions. While the clinical presentation can be very helpful in distinguishing between the causes of STE in some cases, it does not always settle the matter.

How then can the ECG best be used when treating cardiac patients in the early hours of chest pain? *A realistic initial goal is to recognize situations when STE could be the result of an MI or other conditions.* For example, LBBB can very closely simulate the ECG pattern of an anterior wall infarction. However, you need not attempt to determine if the cause of the STE is an infarction or an STE variant. In these instances, simply note the presence of STE, recognize that it could be attributed to an infarct or an STE variant, and bring it to the attention of the emergency department (ED) provider for review. When the patient's clinical presentation is suspicious enough to motivate you to obtain a 12-lead ECG, the presence of an STE variant should prompt an immediate review by the ED provider.

The ED provider can determine if the patient should be worked up as a cardiac patient. Outside the hospital, the paramedic should transmit the ECG for interpretation by an ED provider. If transmission is impossible, objective findings can be relayed via radio or phone. For example, one may state, "There is 4 to 5 mm of STE in V_1 through V_3, and an LBBB pattern is present." Given that information, the ED provider will immediately realize the interpretive predicament and can determine whether the paramedic should proceed with reperfusion therapy screening, aspirin, and multiple intravenous lines.

This approach may seem inappropriate in some ways, but it is not. In fact, sometimes, the phrase "I don't know" is the most intelligent response you can give. In situations where there is insufficient information to make a reasonable interpretation, it is far better to defer to the ED provider than to assign an interpretation without sufficient evidence. Often, the provider will not have an immediate answer either. It may be that only after comparative and serial ECGs are available, cardiac biomarkers are analyzed, and the patient is observed over time that the provider will feel comfortable applying a definitive interpretation. Therefore, do not be disheartened by this predicament. Table 4.2 summarizes the five STE variants discussed in this chapter and how they mimic infarction.

TABLE 4.2	Summary of Five Common ST-Elevation Variants	
Condition	**Infarction Resemblance**	**Recognition**
LVH	• STE in the negatively deflected leads, usually V_1 to V_3	• Add S-wave amplitude in lead V_3 and R-wave amplitude in lead aVL • Suspect LVH if total greater than 20 mm (2 mV) in women and 28 mm (2.8 mV) or more in men
LBBB	• STE in the negatively deflected leads, usually V_1 to V_3 • QS complexes in the negatively deflected leads, usually V_1 to V_3	• QRS complex 120 msec or more • QRS complex produced by supraventricular activity • QS complex or negative terminal force in V_1

Continued

TABLE 4.2   Summary of Five Common ST-Elevation Variants—cont'd

Condition	Infarction Resemblance	Recognition
Ventricular rhythms	• STE in the negatively deflected leads • QS complexes in the negatively deflected leads	• Wide QRS complex following pacer spikes (if noticeable) • Negative terminal force in V_1 (right ventricle paced)
Early repolarization	• STE, particularly in anterior or anterolateral leads • Tall T waves	• Widespread STE with rapidly upsloping (ascending) shape of the initial portion of the ST segment that is typically maximal in leads V_2 to V_5 • Notching at the end of the QRS complex (J point) or slurring on the downstroke of the R wave • Concordant T waves of large amplitude • QRS duration less than 120 msec
Pericarditis	• STE in multiple leads	• STE not in anatomical grouping • STE usually present in leads I, II, III, aVL, aVF, and V_2 through V_6 • Reciprocal ST depression in aVR and V_1 • PR-segment elevation in aVR, with PR-segment depression in other leads • Notching of the J point

LBBB, Left bundle branch block; *LVH*, left ventricular hypertrophy; *msec*, milliseconds; *STE*, ST-elevation.

REFERENCES

Abbas, H., Roomi, S., Ullah, W., Ahmad, A., & Gajanan, G. (2019). Brugada pattern: A comprehensive review on the demographic and clinical spectrum. *BMJ Case Reports, 12*(7), e229829. doi:10.1136/bcr-2019-229829.

Antzelevitch, C., Yan, G., Ackerman, M. J., Borggrefe, M., Corrado, D., Guo, J., Gussak, I., Hasdemir, C., Horie, M., Huikuri, H., Ma, C., Morita, H., Nam, G. B., Sacher, F., Shimizu, W., Viskin, S., & Wilde, A. A. (2017). J-wave syndromes expert consensus conference report: Emerging concepts and gaps in knowledge. *Europace, 19*(4), 665–694.

Goldberger, A. L., Goldberger, Z. D., & Shvilkin, A. (2024). Atrial and ventricular overload/enlargement. In *Goldberger's clinical electrocardiography: A simplified approach* (10th ed., pp. 52–63). Elsevier.

Hancock, E. W., Deal, B. J., Mirvis, D. M., Okin, P., Kligfield, P., & Gettes, L. S. (2009). AHA/ACCF/HRS recommendations for the standardization and interpretation of the electrocardiogram: Part V: Electrocardiogram changes associated with cardiac chamber hypertrophy. *Journal of the American College of Cardiology, 53*(11), 992–1002.

Kusumoto, F. M., Schoenfeld, M. H., Barrett, C., Edgerton, J. R., Ellenbogen, K. A., Gold, M. R., … Varosy, P. D. (2019). 2018 ACC/AHA/HRS guideline on the evaluation and management of patients with bradycardia and cardiac conduction delay. *Heart Rhythm, 16*(9), e128–e226.

Mirvis, D. M., & Goldberger, A. L. (2022). Electrocardiography. In P. Libby, R. O., Bonow, D. L., Mann, G. F., Tomaselli, D. L., Bhatt, & S. D. Solomon (Eds.), *Braunwald's heart disease: A textbook of cardiovascular medicine* (12th ed., pp. 141–174). Elsevier.

Rankinen, J., Haataja, P., Lyytikäinen, L. P., Huhtala, H., Lehtimäki, T., Kähönen, M., … Hernesniemi, J. (2020). Relation of intraventricular conduction delay to risk of new-onset heart failure and structural heart disease in the general population. *International Journal of Cardiology. Heart & Vasculature, 31*, 100639.

Rosso, R., Glikson, E., Belhassen, B., Katz, A., Halkin, A., Steinvil, A., & Viskin, S. (2012). Distinguishing "benign" from "malignant early repolarization": The value of the ST-segment morphology. *Heart Rhythm, 9*(2), 225–229.

Sgarbossa, E. B., Pinski, S. L., Barbagelata, A., Underwood, D. A., Gates, K. B., Topol, E. J., … Wagner, G. S. (1996). Electrocardiographic diagnosis of evolving acute myocardial infarction in the presence of left bundle-branch block. GUSTO-1 (Global Utilization of Streptokinase and Tissue Plasminogen Activator for Occluded Coronary Arteries) Investigators. *New England Journal of Medicine, 334*(8), 481–487.

Smith, S. W., Dodd, K. W., Henry, T. D., Dvorak, D. M., & Pearce, L. A. (2012). Diagnosis of ST-elevation myocardial infarction in the presence of left bundle branch block with the ST-elevation to S-wave ratio in a modified Sgarbossa rule. *Annals of Emergency Medicine, 60*(6), 766–776.

QUICK REVIEW

1. Which of the following is true about the left anterior fascicle?
   a. It is short and thick, and impulse transmission is rarely disrupted.
   b. It is thin and vulnerable to disruptions in electrical impulse transmission.
   c. It relays the impulse to the inferior and posterior portions of the left ventricle.
   d. It receives a dual blood supply from the LAD and the right coronary artery.
   e. It receives its blood supply primarily from septal branches of the LAD artery.
   f. It spreads the electrical impulse to the anterior and lateral portions of the left ventricle.

2. Which of the following are characteristics of a RBBB?
   a. Pathologic Q waves
   b. An rSR' pattern in leads V_1 or V_2
   c. A broad R wave in leads I and V_6
   d. A QRS duration of 120 msec or more if a complete RBBB

3. A complete BBB is characterized by a
   a. QRS measuring 100 to 119 msec.
   b. QRS measuring 120 msec or more.
   c. QT interval measuring less than 440 msec.
   d. PR interval measuring more than 200 msec.

4. Which of the following are characteristics of a left posterior fascicular block?
   a. Right axis deviation
   b. An rS pattern in leads I and aVL
   c. A qR pattern in leads III and aVF
   d. A QRS duration of 120 msec or more

5. Patients experiencing which of the following types of infarctions are most likely to develop a BBB?
   a. Septal
   b. Lateral
   c. Inferior
   d. Inferobasal
   e. Inferolateral
   f. Anteroseptal

6. ER
   a. is associated with an increased incidence of cardiogenic shock.
   b. is an electrocardiographic variant that most often occurs in elderly men.
   c. produces ST-segment depression that is typically seen in the limb leads.
   d. produces an electrocardiographic pattern resembling an anterior infarction.

7. Which of the following ECG changes may be observed with pericarditis?
   a. J-point notching
   b. QRS duration of 120 msec or more
   c. STE that consistently appears in anatomical lead groupings
   d. PR-segment elevation in lead aVR, with reciprocal PR-segment depression in other leads

8. Which ECG characteristics are typically associated with left ventricular hypertrophy?
   a. Right axis deviation
   b. Tall, peaked T waves
   c. PR-segment depression
   d. Increased QRS amplitude
   e. Deeper than normal S waves
   f. ST-segment and T-wave changes

CASE STUDIES

For each of the following case studies, carefully evaluate the description of the patient's clinical presentation, systematically analyze each 12-lead ECG, and formulate a treatment plan based on the information provided.

CASE STUDY 4.1

A 78-year-old man presents with a sudden onset of shortness of breath and "feeling faint." While speaking in sentences of four to five words, he relays that he was using a plunger to clear a clogged toilet when his symptoms began about 45 minutes ago. He denies chest pain. The patient has a history of asthma, for which he takes albuterol and ipratropium bromide. He has no known allergies.

Physical examination reveals the patient is alert, anxious, and oriented to person, place, time, and event. His skin is pink, warm, and dry, and there is no jugular vein distention. Bilateral inspiratory and expiratory wheezing is present. His blood pressure is 170/110 mm Hg, heart rate 100 beats/min, ventilations 24/min, and SpO_2 90% on room air.

The patient has been placed on a cardiac monitor, and supplemental oxygen is being administered. Vascular access has been established, and a 12-lead ECG has been obtained (Fig. 4.22). Review the patient's ECG and describe your initial interventions for this patient.

Fig. **4.22**

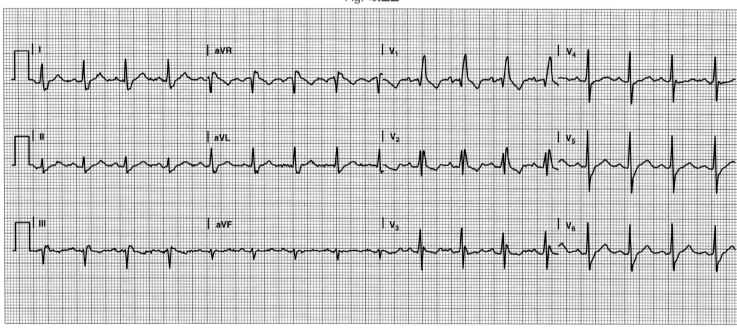

CASE STUDY 4.2

A 78-year-old man presents with a sudden onset of substernal chest pain and shortness of breath that began 3 hours ago while at rest. He rates his pain 9/10 and says it radiates to his left arm and back. The patient had a coronary artery bypass graft 4 years ago.

The patient regularly takes at least 20 medications, which he has brought with him. He is allergic to codeine. Physical examination reveals that the patient is alert, anxious, and oriented to person, place, time, and event. His skin is pink, warm, and moist, and his breath sounds are clear. His SpO$_2$ is 98% on room air, blood pressure 178/82 mm Hg, pulse 120 beats/min, and ventilations 26/min.

The patient has been placed on a cardiac monitor, vascular access has been established, and a 12-lead ECG has been obtained (Fig. 4.23). Review the patient's ECG and describe your initial interventions for this patient.

Fig. **4.23**

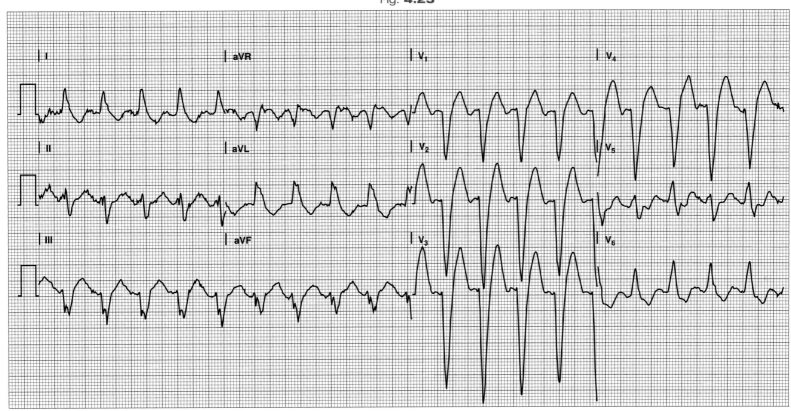

ANSWERS

1. **B, E, F.** The anterior fascicle receives its blood supply from septal branches of the LAD. It spreads the electrical impulse to the anterior and lateral portions of the left ventricle. This fascicle is thin and vulnerable to disruptions in electrical impulse transmission. In contrast, impulse transmission in the posterior fascicle is rarely disrupted because it is short, thick, and receives a dual blood supply from the LAD and the right coronary artery. This fascicle relays the impulse to the inferior and posterior portions of the left ventricle.

2. **B, D.** An rsr', rsR', rSR', or (rarely) a qR pattern in leads V_1 or V_2 are characteristic of RBBB. Additional characteristics include an S wave of greater duration than the R wave or more than 40 msec in leads I and V6, and a QRS duration of 120 msec or more if a complete RBBB; a QRS duration between 110 and 119 msec if incomplete.

3. **B.** A complete BBB has a QRS complex duration of 120 msec or more and, if incomplete, a QRS duration between 110 and 119 msec.

4. **A, B, C.** The ECG characteristics of left posterior fascicular block include right axis deviation, an rS pattern in leads I and aVL, a qR pattern in leads III and aVF, and a QRS duration of less than 120 msec.

5. **A, F.** Because the LAD artery supplies much of the bundle branches, patients experiencing septal and anteroseptal infarctions are most likely to develop BBB.

6. **D.** ER is a normal electrocardiographic variant that produces a pattern resembling an anterior or anterolateral infarction on the ECGs of healthy asymptomatic patients. It is most often seen in young athletic individuals. ER produces STE that is generally maximal in leads V_2 to V_5.

7. **A, D.** ECG changes that may be observed with pericarditis include J-point notching, diffuse STE that is not strictly grouped into anatomically contiguous leads, and PR-segment elevation in lead aVR, with reciprocal PR-segment depression in other leads.

8. **D, F.** Left ventricular hypertrophy is primarily recognized on the ECG by increased QRS amplitude accompanied by changes in the ST segment and T wave. Typically, R waves in leads facing the left ventricle (i.e., I, aVL, V_5, and V_6) are taller than normal, and S waves in leads V_1 and V_2 are deeper than normal.

INTERPRETATION OF CASE STUDIES

CASE STUDY 4.1

Although this patient's symptoms are likely to be respiratory in origin, shortness of breath is also an anginal equivalent. Allow the patient to assume a position of comfort and measure his peak expiratory flow rate. Administer a bronchodilator and an inhaled corticosteroid and reassess. The patient's 12-lead ECG shows sinus tachycardia with a RBBB but no evidence of STEMI at this time.

The patient's symptoms resolved over a period of 2 hours in the ED. After evaluating the results of his chest radiograph, a second 12-lead ECG, and laboratory studies, the patient was discharged home with the addition of an inhaled corticosteroid to his asthma therapy regimen.

CASE STUDY 4.2

The patient's 12-lead ECG shows ECG changes consistent with an anteroseptal STEMI; however, an LBBB is present. LBBB can cause STE and T-wave changes, confounding the ECG diagnosis of STEMI. While none of the modified Sgarbossa criteria have been met, the shape of the ST segments here makes STEMI a strong consideration.

Give aspirin as soon as possible if not already done and if there are no contraindications. Quickly screen the patient for indications and contraindications to fibrinolytic therapy and percutaneous coronary intervention. At the same time, administer nitroglycerin (NTG) to address the patient's ischemic chest discomfort. Closely monitor the patient's vital signs and ECG after each dose. Select a reperfusion strategy, obtain a portable chest radiograph, and draw initial laboratory studies.

After one sublingual NTG tablet, the patient rated his chest pain 8/10. After a second tablet, 7/10, and after a third, 4/10. The patient was then given intravenous morphine and moved to the cardiac catheterization laboratory.

Practice ECGs

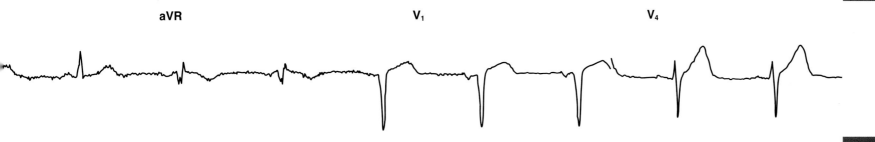

LEARNING OBJECTIVES

After reading this chapter, you should be able to:

1. Develop a systematic approach for infarct recognition on the electrocardiogram (ECG).
2. Gain familiarity with 12-lead ECG interpretation.

12-LEAD ANALYSIS

We began discussing the approach to reviewing a 12-lead ECG in Chapter 3. This chapter expands that approach to include ST-elevation (STE) variants and the patient's clinical presentation.

1. Identify the rate and underlying rhythm.
2. Analyze waveforms, segments, and intervals. Examine each lead (except aVR), looking for the following:
   - *Pathologic Q waves.* Recall that a pathologic Q wave is abnormally wide and deep. Suspect an infarction when Q waves appear in several leads or lead groups, are more than 0.04 second, or are associated with ST or T-wave changes in the same leads.
   - *R-wave progression.* Recall that when viewing the chest leads in a normal heart, the R wave typically becomes taller (i.e., increases in amplitude), and the S wave becomes smaller as the electrode is moved from right to left. In the area of leads V_3 and V_4, the amplitude of the R wave should begin to exceed the amplitude of the S wave and then gradually become smaller again through V_6. Use the phrase *poor R-wave progression* to describe R waves that decrease in size from V_1 to V_4.
   - *ST-segment displacement.* Looking at the J point, determine if STE or ST-segment depression is present.
   - *T-wave changes.* Examine the T waves for changes in orientation, shape, and size. Note if they are tall, peaked, inverted, biphasic, or notched.
3. Examine for evidence of acute coronary syndrome (ACS). If ST-segment displacement is present, assess the areas of ischemia or injury by evaluating lead groupings.
4. Ascertain if an STE variant is present that may account for ECG changes (Box 5.1).
   - Use one of several available formulas to rule out left ventricular hypertrophy (LVH) as a possible cause of STE.
   - Bundle branch blocks (BBBs) and ventricular rhythms can cause a wide QRS and mimic the infarct pattern on the ECG. However, if the QRS is of normal duration (110 milliseconds [msec] or less), no *complete* BBB or ventricular rhythm exists, and you can scratch BBB and ventricular rhythms from the list of STE variants.

Box **5.1**	Examples of ST-Elevation Variants

- LVH
- LBBB
- Ventricular rhythms
- ER
- Pericarditis

- Early repolarization (ER) and pericarditis can also cause STE, mimicking an infarct pattern on the ECG. However, neither ER nor pericarditis is particularly good at causing reciprocal changes. Therefore, if STE is present on the ECG and clear, obvious, reciprocal changes are present, it is reasonable to scratch ER and pericarditis from the list of possible causes of STE.
- The presence of an STE variant does not rule out myocardial infarction (MI). Sometimes the ECG will show STE *and* meet the criteria for LVH. In this situation, LVH may be the cause of the STE. However, it is also possible that the patient may have an enlarged left ventricle *and* simultaneously have a clot in a coronary artery. Similarly, a patient may have a BBB *and* be experiencing an MI. In such cases, a physician should be consulted.

5. Estimate the QRS axis using leads I and aVF.
6. Interpret your findings. Categorize the 12-lead ECG into one of the following groups: (1) STE, (2) ST-segment depression, or (3) normal or nondiagnostic ECG.

Clinical Presentation

Discovering the patient's clinical presentation is a priority. However, including the clinical presentation at this point does not imply that it is the first time you should obtain patient information. Rather, it is assumed that you will already have obtained the patient's relevant subjective and objective information. The specific inclusion of the clinical presentation is included here to emphasize the importance of integrating the clinical presentation into the ECG interpretation. When incorporating the clinical picture into the ECG interpretation, remember that not all patients experiencing an ACS will present with substernal chest pain. Therefore, a high index of suspicion is always warranted, especially when treating women, individuals with diabetes, or older adults.

Complicating the effort to recognize infarction is the fact that only a minority of nontraumatic chest pain results from infarction. Causes of noninfarction chest pain include pericarditis, aneurysm, musculoskeletal pain, several pulmonary conditions, gastrointestinal disorders, and various emotional and psychological states. Clearly, the task of early infarct recognition can be challenging. Ultimately, it is the provider's task to differentiate infarction from other conditions.

PRACTICE ECGs

Our interpretation of each of the following practice ECGs is included at the end of this chapter. Please note that the interpretation of each lead and tracing includes only the material discussed in this text. Therefore, experienced electrocardiographers will recognize some conditions or findings not listed in the interpretation.

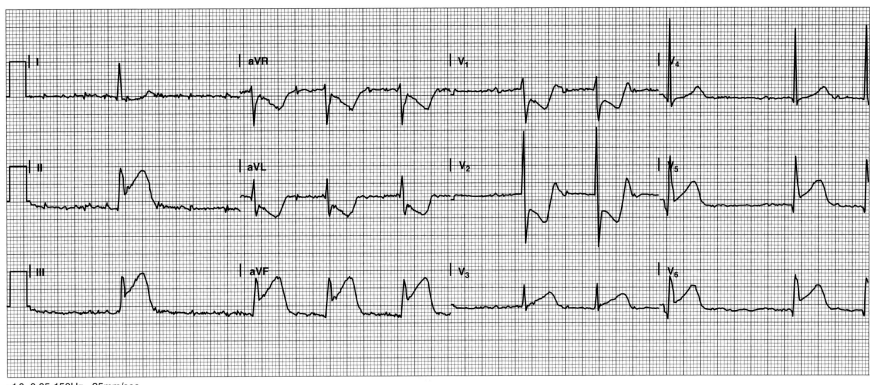

Fig. **5.1**

x1.0 0.05-150Hz   25mm/sec

Rate and rhythm? _____ Pathologic Q waves? _____

STE? _____ ST depression? _____ T-wave changes? _____

Reciprocal changes? _____ STE variant present? _____ Axis? _____

Interpretation: _____

Inferior: II, III, aVF | **Septum: V_1, V_2** | **Anterior: V_3, V_4** | **Lateral: I, aVL, V_5, V_6**

Fig. **5.2**

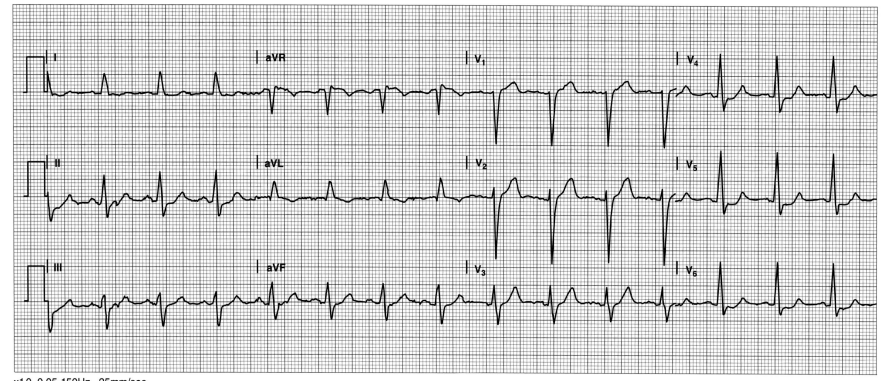

x1.0 0.05-150Hz   25mm/sec

Rate and rhythm? _____ Pathologic Q waves? _____

STE? _____ ST depression? _____ T-wave changes? _____

Reciprocal changes? _____ STE variant present? _____ Axis? _____

Interpretation: _____

Inferior: II, III, aVF | Septum: V$_1$, V$_2$ | Anterior: V$_3$, V$_4$ | Lateral: I, aVL, V$_5$, V$_6$

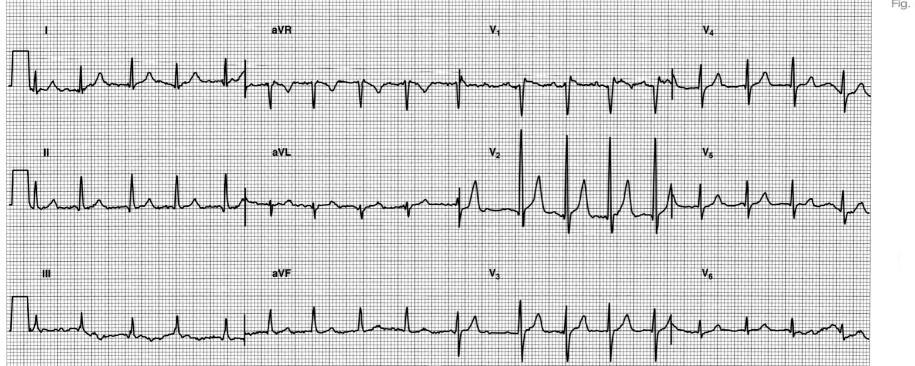

Fig. **5.3**

Rate and rhythm? _____ Pathologic Q waves? _____

STE? _____ ST depression? _____ T-wave changes? _____

Reciprocal changes? _____ STE variant present? _____ Axis? _____

Interpretation: _____

Inferior: II, III, aVF | Septum: V_1, V_2 | Anterior: V_3, V_4 | Lateral: I, aVL, V_5, V_6

Fig. **5.4**

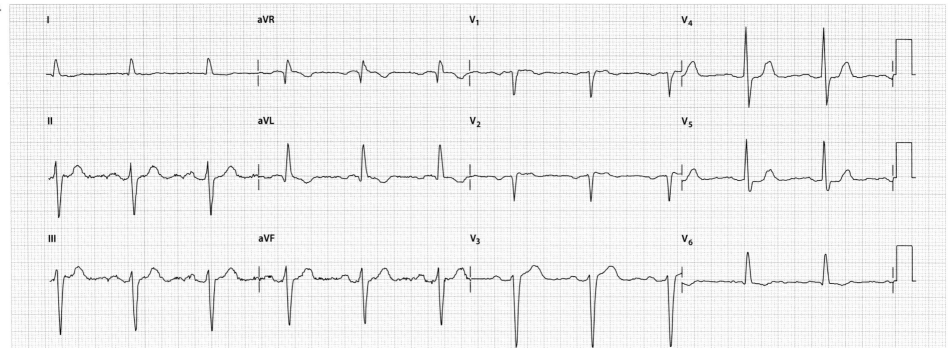

Rate and rhythm? _____ Pathologic Q waves? _____

STE? _____ ST depression? _____ T-wave changes? _____

Reciprocal changes? _____ STE variant present? _____ Axis? _____

Interpretation: _____

Inferior: II, III, aVF | Septum: V₁, V₂ | Anterior: V₃, V₄ | Lateral: I, aVL, V₅, V₆

Fig. **5.5**

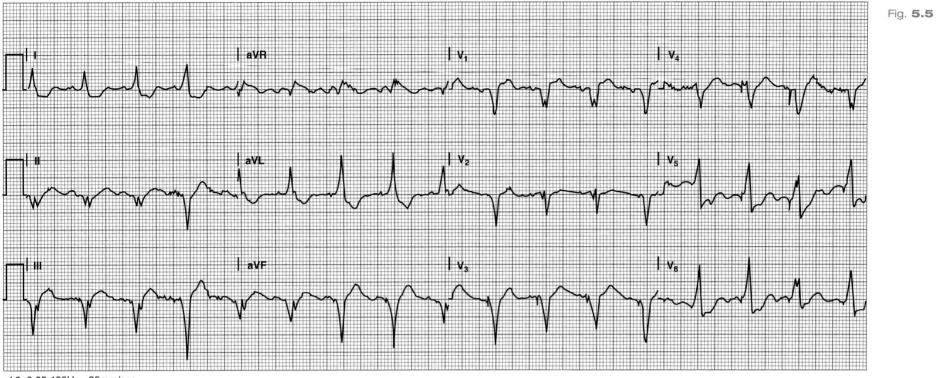

x1.0 0.05-150Hz 25mm/sec

Rate and rhythm? _____ Pathologic Q waves? _____

STE? _____ ST depression? _____ T-wave changes? _____

Reciprocal changes? _____ STE variant present? _____ Axis? _____

Interpretation: _____

Inferior: II, III, aVF | Septum: V$_1$, V$_2$ | Anterior: V$_3$, V$_4$ | Lateral: I, aVL, V$_5$, V$_6$

Fig. **5.6**

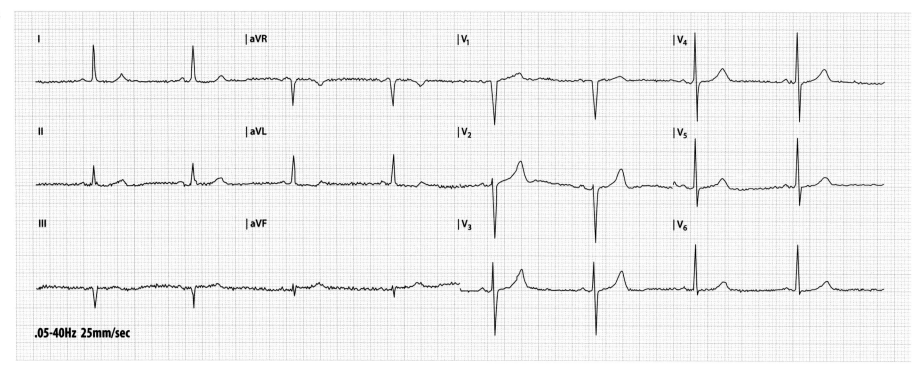

.05-40Hz 25mm/sec

Rate and rhythm? _____ Pathologic Q waves? _____

STE? _____ ST depression? _____ T-wave changes? _____

Reciprocal changes? _____ STE variant present? _____ Axis? _____

Interpretation: _____

Inferior: II, III, aVF | Septum: V₁, V₂ | Anterior: V₃, V₄ | Lateral: I, aVL, V₅, V₆

Fig. **5.7**

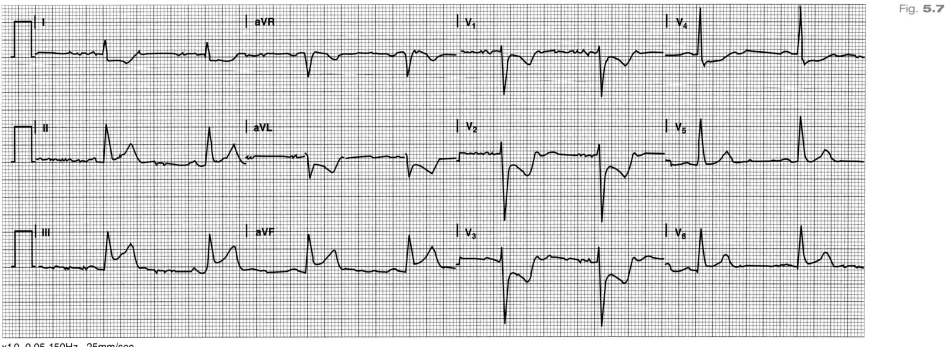

x1.0 0.05-150Hz 25mm/sec

Rate and rhythm? _____ Pathologic Q waves? _____

STE? _____ ST depression? _____ T-wave changes? _____

Reciprocal changes? _____ STE variant present? _____ Axis? _____

Interpretation: _____

Inferior: II, III, aVF | Septum: V₁, V₂ | Anterior: V₃, V₄ | **Lateral: I, aVL, V₅, V₆**

Fig.  **5.8**

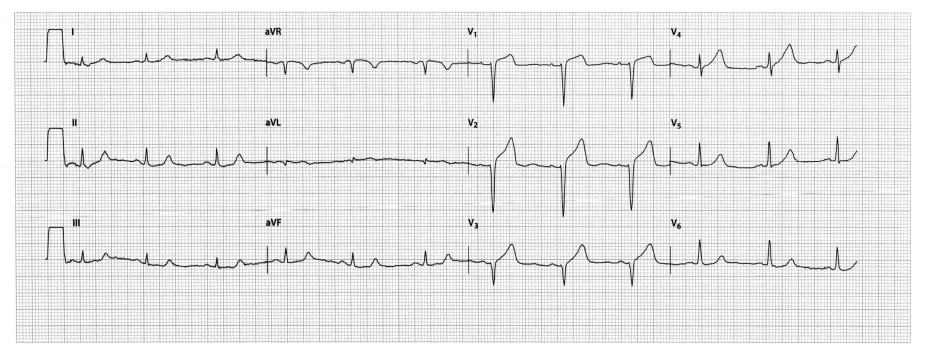

Rate and rhythm? _____ Pathologic Q waves? _____

STE? _____ ST depression? _____ T-wave changes? _____

Reciprocal changes? _____ STE variant present? _____ Axis? _____

Interpretation: _____

Inferior: II, III, aVF | **Septum: V₁, V₂** | **Anterior: V₃, V₄** | **Lateral: I, aVL, V₅, V₆**

Fig. **5.9**

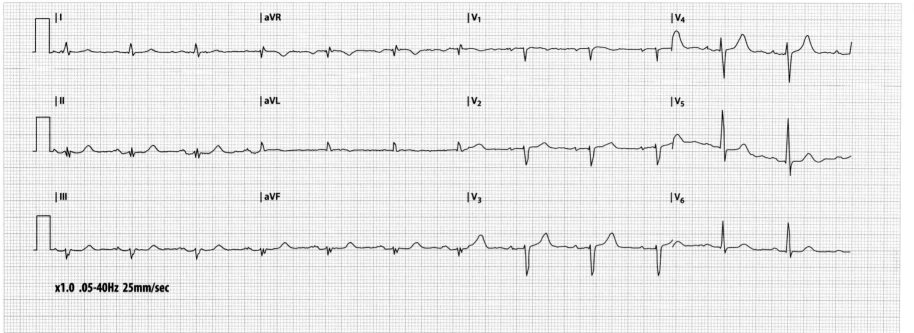

x1.0 .05-40Hz 25mm/sec

Rate and rhythm? _____ Pathologic Q waves? _____

STE? _____ ST depression? _____ T-wave changes? _____

Reciprocal changes? _____ STE variant present? _____ Axis? _____

Interpretation: _____

Inferior: II, III, aVF | Septum: V₁, V₂ | Anterior: V₃, V₄ | **Lateral: I, aVL, V₅, V₆**

Fig. **5.10**

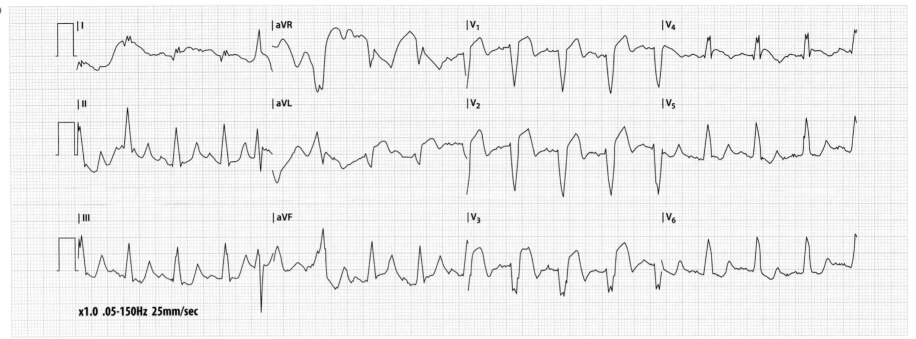

x1.0 .05-150Hz 25mm/sec

Rate and rhythm? _____ Pathologic Q waves? _____

STE? _____ ST depression? _____ T-wave changes? _____

Reciprocal changes? _____ STE variant present? _____ Axis? _____

Interpretation: _____

Inferior: II, III, aVF | Septum: V_1, V_2 | Anterior: V_3, V_4 | Lateral: I, aVL, V_5, V_6

Fig. **5.11**

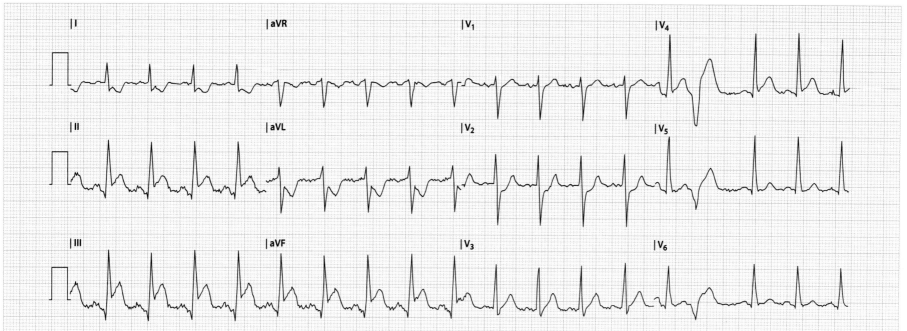

Rate and rhythm? _____ Pathologic Q waves? _____

STE? _____ ST depression? _____ T-wave changes? _____

Reciprocal changes? _____ STE variant present? _____ Axis? _____

Interpretation: _____

Inferior: II, III, aVF | Septum: V₁, V₂ | Anterior: V₃, V₄ | **Lateral: I, aVL, V₅, V₆**

Fig. **5.12**

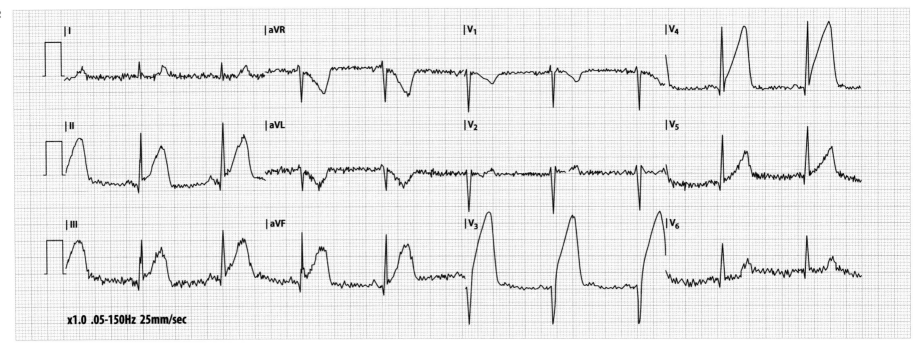

x1.0 .05-150Hz 25mm/sec

Rate and rhythm? _____ Pathologic Q waves? _____

STE? _____ ST depression? _____ T-wave changes? _____

Reciprocal changes? _____ STE variant present? _____ Axis? _____

Interpretation: _____

Inferior: II, III, aVF | Septum: V$_1$, V$_2$ | Anterior: V$_3$, V$_4$ | Lateral: I, aVL, V$_5$, V$_6$

Fig. 5.13

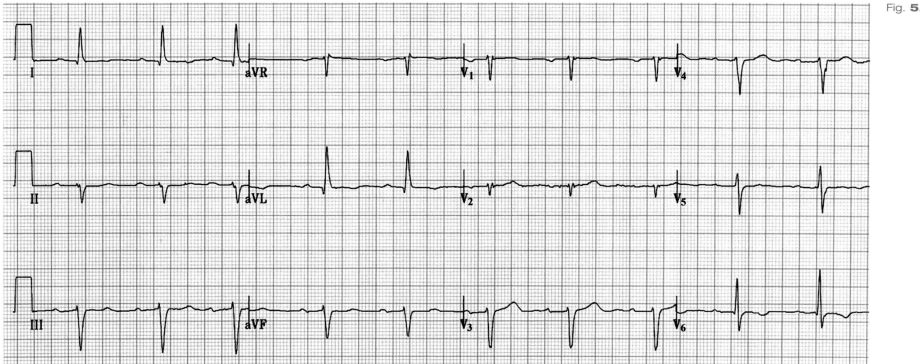

Rate and rhythm? _____ Pathologic Q waves? _____

STE? _____ ST depression? _____ T-wave changes? _____

Reciprocal changes? _____ STE variant present? _____ Axis? _____

Interpretation: _____

Inferior: II, III, aVF | Septum: V₁, V₂ | Anterior: V₃, V₄ | **Lateral: I, aVL, V₅, V₆**

Fig. 5.14

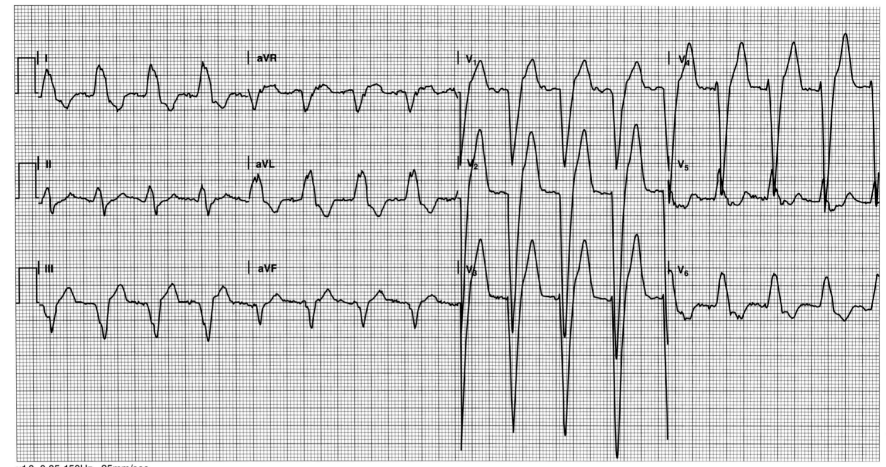

x1.0 0.05-150Hz 25mm/sec

Rate and rhythm? _____ Pathologic Q waves? _____

STE? _____ ST depression? _____ T-wave changes? _____

Reciprocal changes? _____ STE variant present? _____ Axis? _____

Interpretation: _____

Inferior: II, III, aVF | Septum: V₁, V₂ | Anterior: V₃, V₄ | Lateral: I, aVL, V₅, V₆

Fig. **5.15**

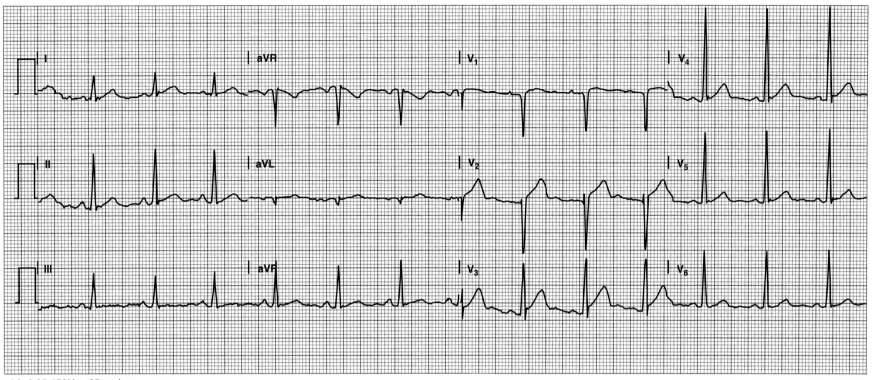

x1.0 0.05-150Hz 25mm/sec

Rate and rhythm? _____ Pathologic Q waves? _____

STE? _____ ST depression? _____ T-wave changes? _____

Reciprocal changes? _____ STE variant present? _____ Axis? _____

Interpretation: _____

Inferior: II, III, aVF | Septum: V₁, V₂ | Anterior: V₃, V₄ | **Lateral: I, aVL, V₅, V₆**

Fig. **5.16**

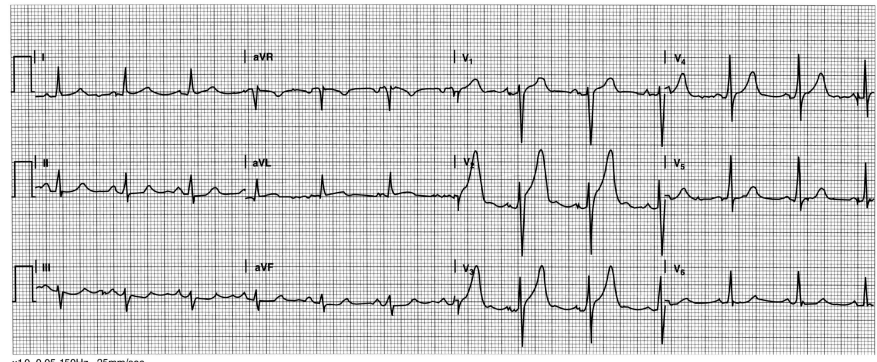

x1.0 0.05-150Hz   25mm/sec

Rate and rhythm? _____ Pathologic Q waves? _____

STE? _____ ST depression? _____ T-wave changes? _____

Reciprocal changes? _____ STE variant present? _____ Axis? _____

Interpretation: _____

Inferior: II, III, aVF | Septum: V₁, V₂ | Anterior: V₃, V₄ | Lateral: I, aVL, V₅, V₆

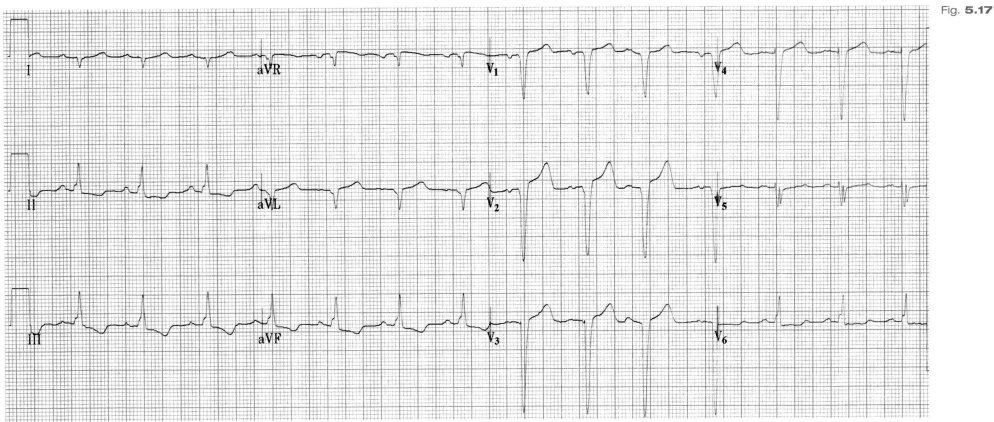

Fig. **5.17**

Rate and rhythm? _____ Pathologic Q waves? _____

STE? _____ ST depression? _____ T-wave changes? _____

Reciprocal changes? _____ STE variant present? _____ Axis? _____

Interpretation: _____

Inferior: II, III, aVF | Septum: V₁, V₂ | Anterior: V₃, V₄ | Lateral: I, aVL, V₅, V₆

Fig. **5.18**

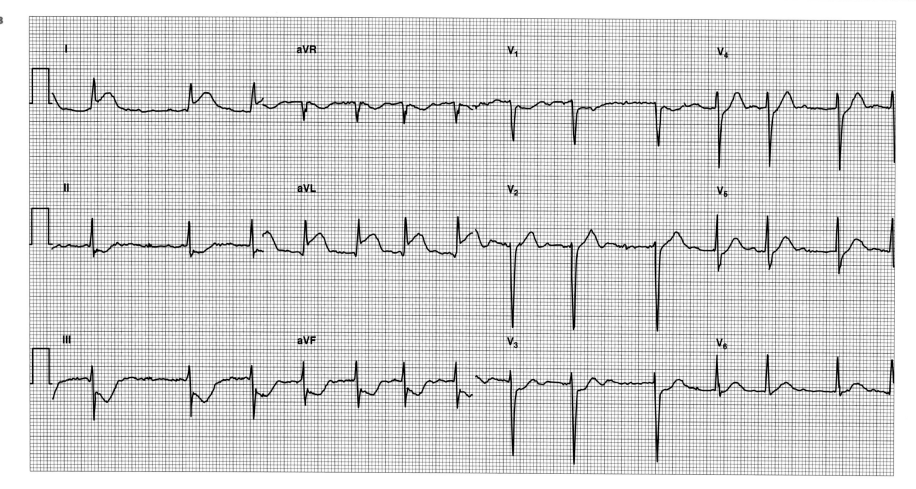

Rate and rhythm? _____ Pathologic Q waves? _____

STE? _____ ST depression? _____ T-wave changes? _____

Reciprocal changes? _____ STE variant present? _____ Axis? _____

Interpretation: _____

Inferior: II, III, aVF | **Septum: V₁, V₂** | **Anterior: V₃, V₄** | **Lateral: I, aVL, V₅, V₆**

Fig. **5.19**

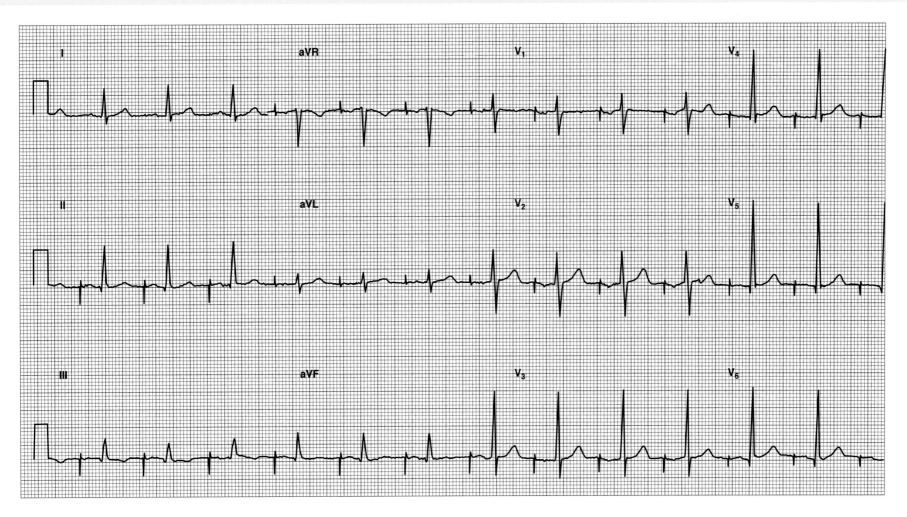

Rate and rhythm? _____ Pathologic Q waves? _____

STE? _____ ST depression? _____ T-wave changes? _____

Reciprocal changes? _____ STE variant present? _____ Axis? _____

Interpretation: _____

Inferior: II, III, aVF | Septum: V₁, V₂ | Anterior: V₃, V₄ | **Lateral: I, aVL, V₅, V₆**

Fig. **5.20**

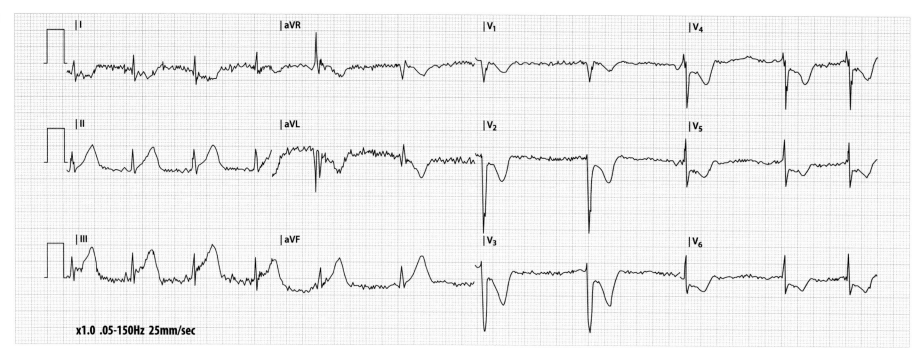

x1.0 .05-150Hz 25mm/sec

Rate and rhythm? _____ Pathologic Q waves? _____

STE? _____ ST depression? _____ T-wave changes? _____

Reciprocal changes? _____ STE variant present? _____ Axis? _____

Interpretation: _____

Inferior: II, III, aVF | Septum: V$_1$, V$_2$ | Anterior: V$_3$, V$_4$ | **Lateral: I, aVL, V$_5$, V$_6$**

Fig. **5.21**

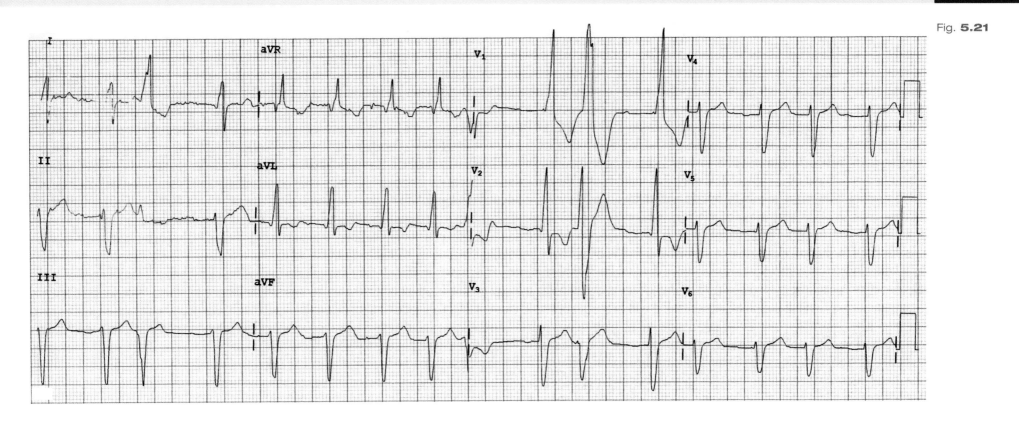

Rate and rhythm? _____ Pathologic Q waves? _____

STE? _____ ST depression? _____ T-wave changes? _____

Reciprocal changes? _____ STE variant present? _____ Axis? _____

Interpretation: _____

Inferior: II, III, aVF | Septum: V₁, V₂ | Anterior: V₃, V₄ | Lateral: I, aVL, V₅, V₆

Fig. **5.22**

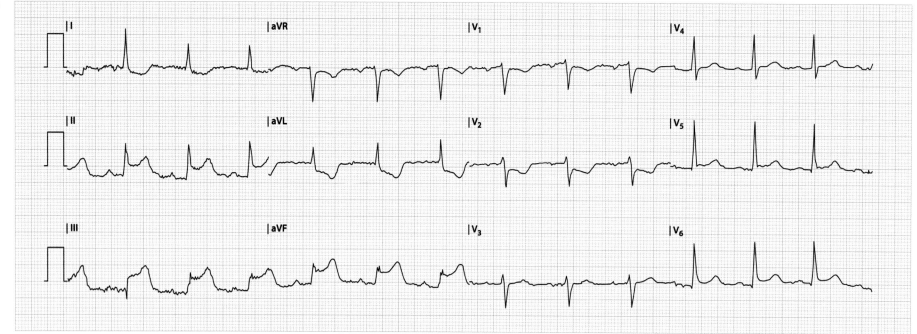

Rate and rhythm? _____ Pathologic Q waves? _____

STE? _____ ST depression? _____ T-wave changes? _____

Reciprocal changes? _____ STE variant present? _____ Axis? _____

Interpretation: _____

Inferior: II, III, aVF | Septum: V_1, V_2 | Anterior: V_3, V_4 | Lateral: I, aVL, V_5, V_6

Fig. **5.23**

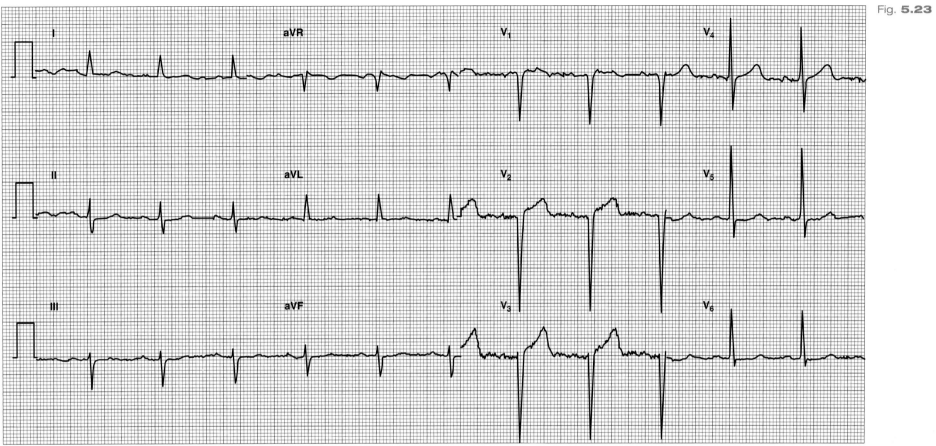

Rate and rhythm? _____ Pathologic Q waves? _____

STE? _____ ST depression? _____ T-wave changes? _____

Reciprocal changes? _____ STE variant present? _____ Axis? _____

Interpretation: _____

Inferior: II, III, aVF | Septum: V₁, V₂ | Anterior: V₃, V₄ | **Lateral: I, aVL, V₅, V₆**

Fig. **5.24**

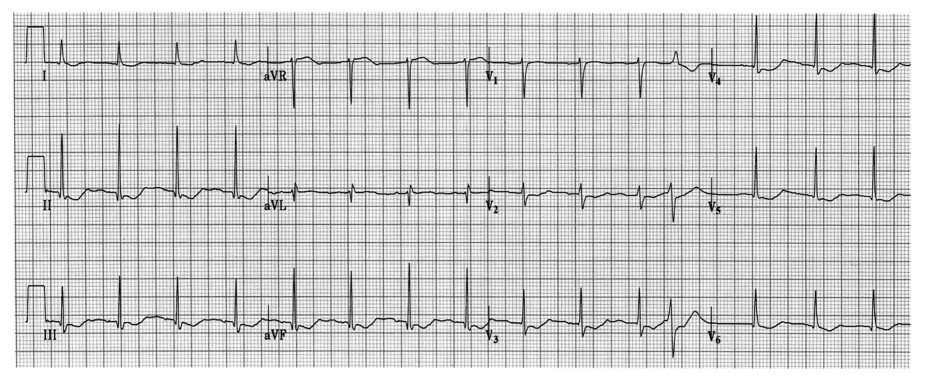

Rate and rhythm? _____ Pathologic Q waves? _____

STE? _____ ST depression? _____ T-wave changes? _____

Reciprocal changes? _____ STE variant present? _____ Axis? _____

Interpretation: _____

Inferior: II, III, aVF | Septum: V₁, V₂ | Anterior: V₃, V₄ | **Lateral: I, aVL, V₅, V₆**

Fig. **5.25**

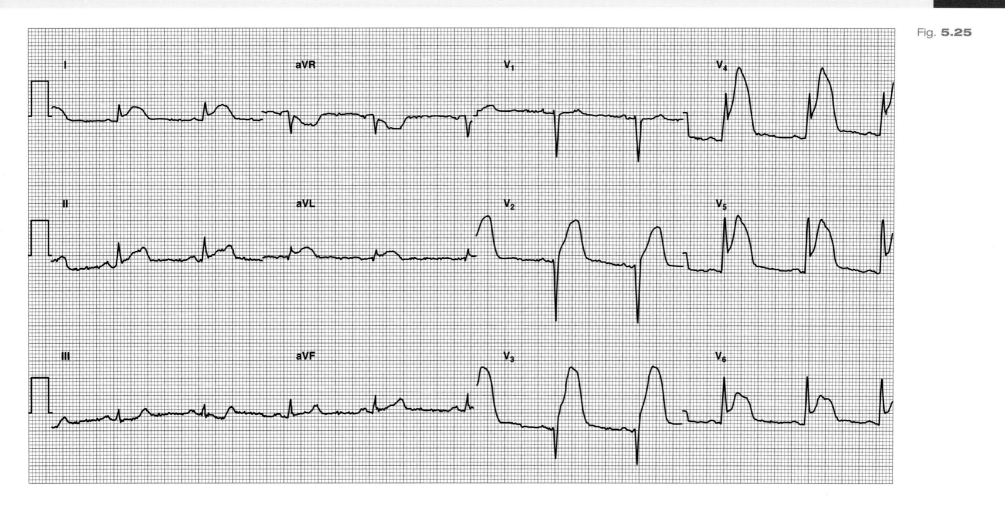

Rate and rhythm? _____ Pathologic Q waves? _____

STE? _____ ST depression? _____ T-wave changes? _____

Reciprocal changes? _____ STE variant present? _____ Axis? _____

Interpretation: _____

Inferior: II, III, aVF | **Septum: V₁, V₂** | **Anterior: V₃, V₄** | **Lateral: I, aVL, V₅, V₆**

Fig. **5.26**

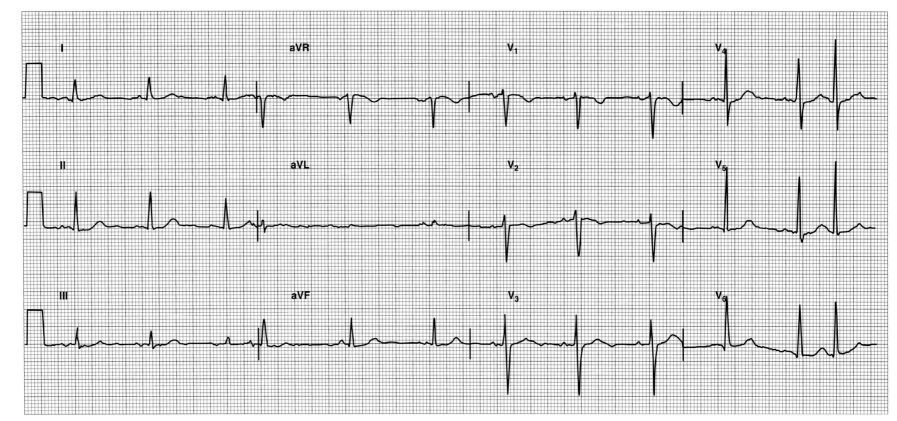

Rate and rhythm? _____ Pathologic Q waves? _____

STE? _____ ST depression? _____ T-wave changes? _____

Reciprocal changes? _____ STE variant present? _____ Axis? _____

Interpretation: _____

Inferior: II, III, aVF | Septum: V$_1$, V$_2$ | Anterior: V$_3$, V$_4$ | **Lateral: I, aVL, V$_5$, V$_6$**

Fig. **5.27**

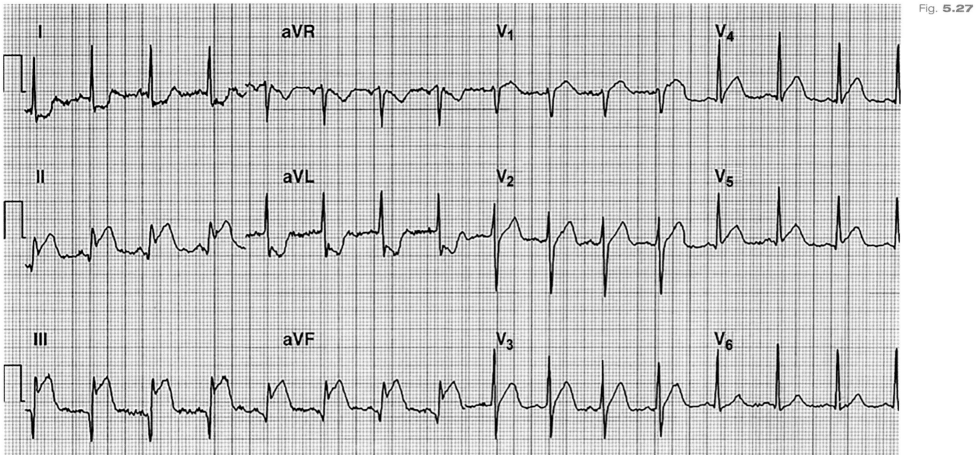

Rate and rhythm? _____ Pathologic Q waves? _____

STE? _____ ST depression? _____ T-wave changes? _____

Reciprocal changes? _____ STE variant present? _____ Axis? _____

Interpretation: _____

Inferior: II, III, aVF | Septum: V₁, V₂ | Anterior: V₃, V₄ | Lateral: I, aVL, V₅, V₆

Fig. **5.28**

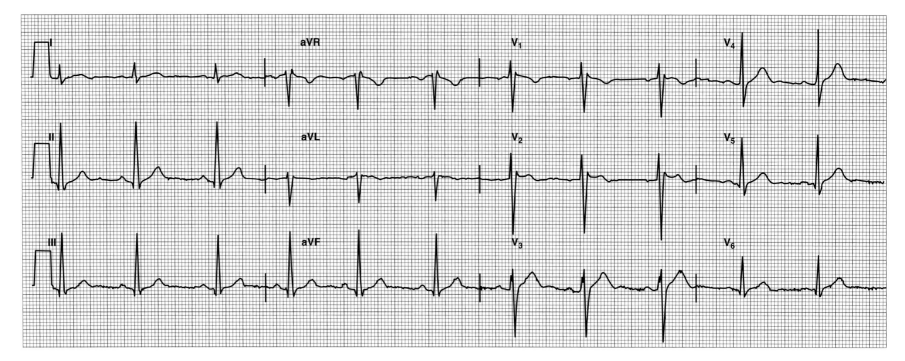

Rate and rhythm? _____ Pathologic Q waves? _____

STE? _____ ST depression? _____ T-wave changes? _____

Reciprocal changes? _____ STE variant present? _____ Axis? _____

Interpretation: _____

Inferior: II, III, aVF | **Septum: V$_1$, V$_2$** | **Anterior: V$_3$, V$_4$** | **Lateral: I, aVL, V$_5$, V$_6$**

Fig. **5.29**

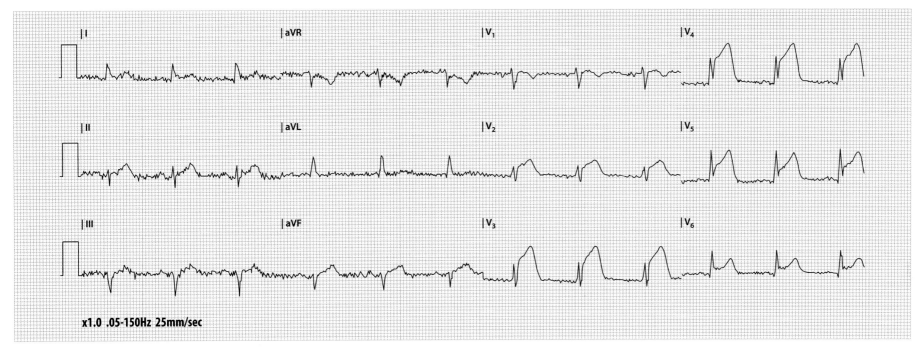

x1.0 .05-150Hz 25mm/sec

Rate and rhythm? _____ Pathologic Q waves? _____

STE? _____ ST depression? _____ T-wave changes? _____

Reciprocal changes? _____ STE variant present? _____ Axis? _____

Interpretation: _____

Inferior: II, III, aVF　|　**Septum: V₁, V₂**　|　**Anterior: V₃, V₄**　|　**Lateral: I, aVL, V₅, V₆**

Fig. **5.30**

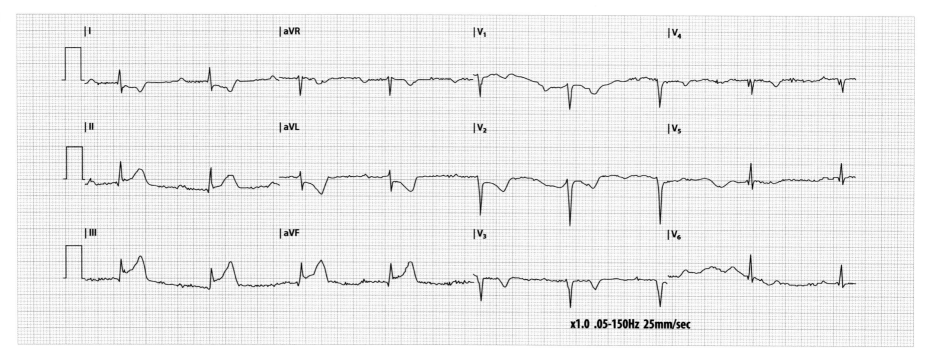

x1.0 .05-150Hz 25mm/sec

Rate and rhythm? _____ Pathologic Q waves? _____

STE? _____ ST depression? _____ T-wave changes? _____

Reciprocal changes? _____ STE variant present? _____ Axis? _____

Interpretation: _____

Inferior: II, III, aVF | Septum: V$_1$, V$_2$ | Anterior: V$_3$, V$_4$ | Lateral: I, aVL, V$_5$, V$_6$

Fig. **5.31**

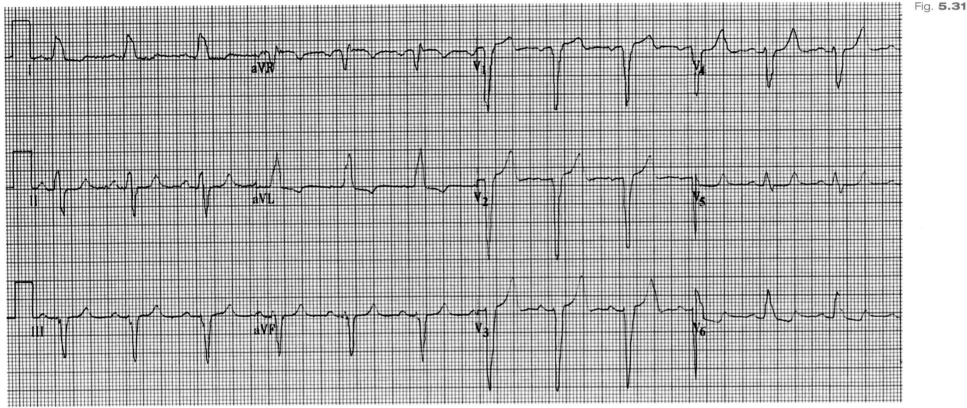

Rate and rhythm? _____ Pathologic Q waves? _____

STE? _____ ST depression? _____ T-wave changes? _____

Reciprocal changes? _____ STE variant present? _____ Axis? _____

Interpretation: _____

Inferior: II, III, aVF | **Septum: V₁, V₂** | **Anterior: V₃, V₄** | **Lateral: I, aVL, V₅, V₆**

Fig. **5.32**

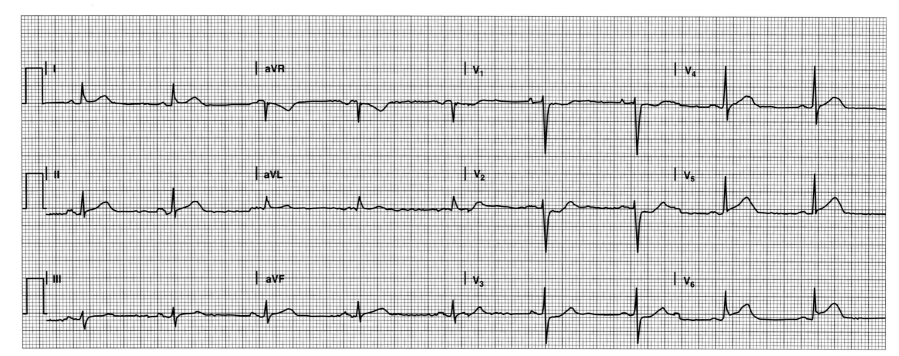

Rate and rhythm? _____ Pathologic Q waves? _____

STE? _____ ST depression? _____ T-wave changes? _____

Reciprocal changes? _____ STE variant present? _____ Axis? _____

Interpretation: _____

Inferior: II, III, aVF | **Septum: V₁, V₂** | **Anterior: V₃, V₄** | **Lateral: I, aVL, V₅, V₆**

Fig. **5.33**

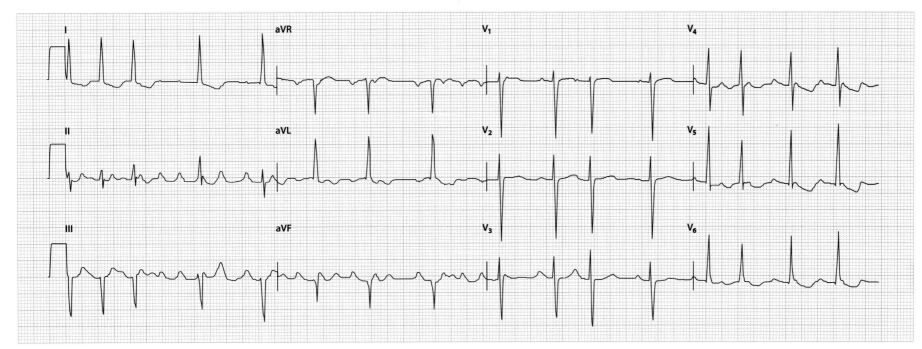

Rate and rhythm? _____ Pathologic Q waves? _____

STE? _____ ST depression? _____ T-wave changes? _____

Reciprocal changes? _____ STE variant present? _____ Axis? _____

Interpretation: _____

Inferior: II, III, aVF | Septum: V₁, V₂ | Anterior: V₃, V₄ | Lateral: I, aVL, V₅, V₆

Fig. **5.34**

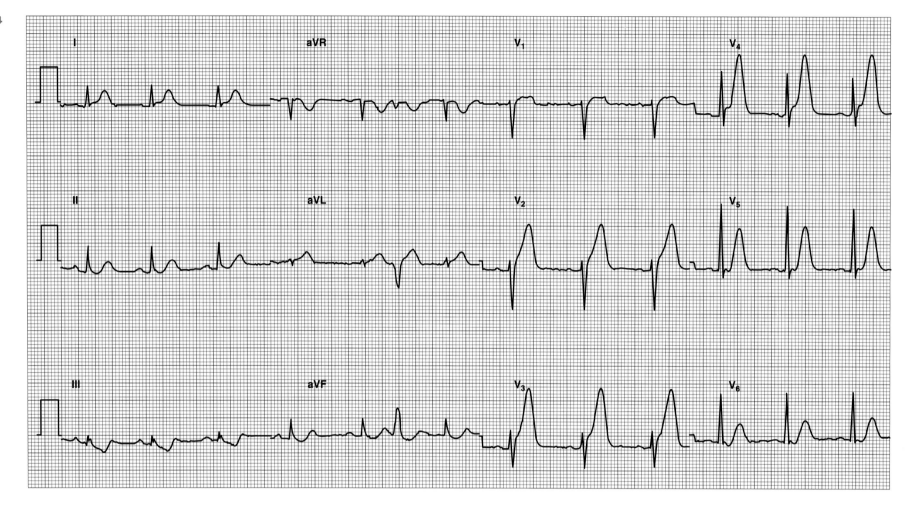

Rate and rhythm? _____ Pathologic Q waves? _____

STE? _____ ST depression? _____ T-wave changes? _____

Reciprocal changes? _____ STE variant present? _____ Axis? _____

Interpretation: _____

Inferior: II, III, aVF | Septum: V₁, V₂ | Anterior: V₃, V₄ | **Lateral: I, aVL, V₅, V₆**

Fig. **5.35**

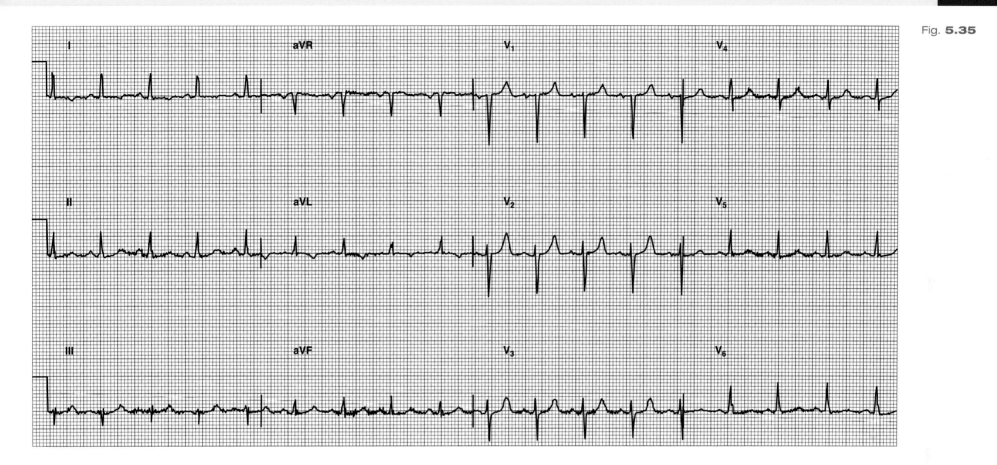

Rate and rhythm? _____ Pathologic Q waves? _____

STE? _____ ST depression? _____ T-wave changes? _____

Reciprocal changes? _____ STE variant present? _____ Axis? _____

Interpretation: _____

Inferior: II, III, aVF | Septum: V₁, V₂ | Anterior: V₃, V₄ | Lateral: I, aVL, V₅, V₆

Fig. 5.36

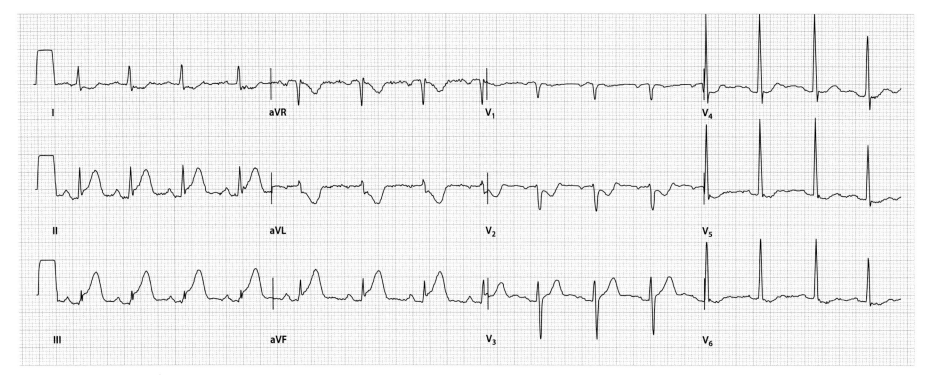

Rate and rhythm? _____ Pathologic Q waves? _____

STE? _____ ST depression? _____ T-wave changes? _____

Reciprocal changes? _____ STE variant present? _____ Axis? _____

Interpretation: _____

Inferior: II, III, aVF | Septum: V$_1$, V$_2$ | Anterior: V$_3$, V$_4$ | Lateral: I, aVL, V$_5$, V$_6$

Fig. **5.37**

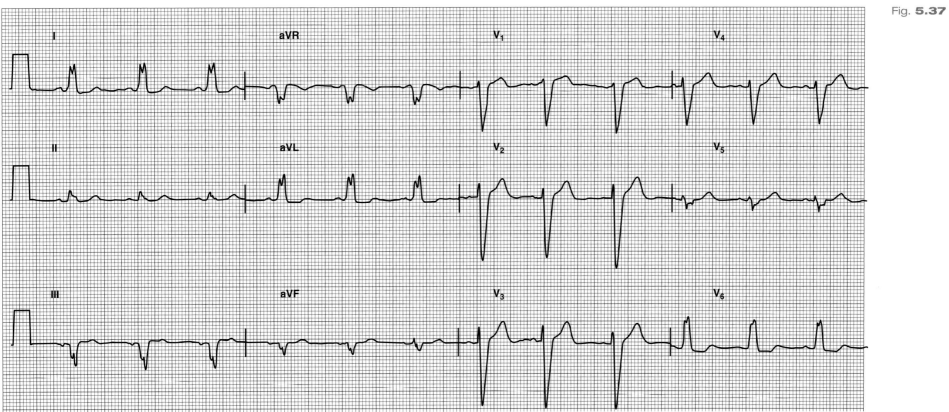

Rate and rhythm? _____ Pathologic Q waves? _____

STE? _____ ST depression? _____ T-wave changes? _____

Reciprocal changes? _____ STE variant present? _____ Axis? _____

Interpretation: _____

Inferior: II, III, aVF | Septum: V$_1$, V$_2$ | Anterior: V$_3$, V$_4$ | Lateral: I, aVL, V$_5$, V$_6$

Fig. 5.38

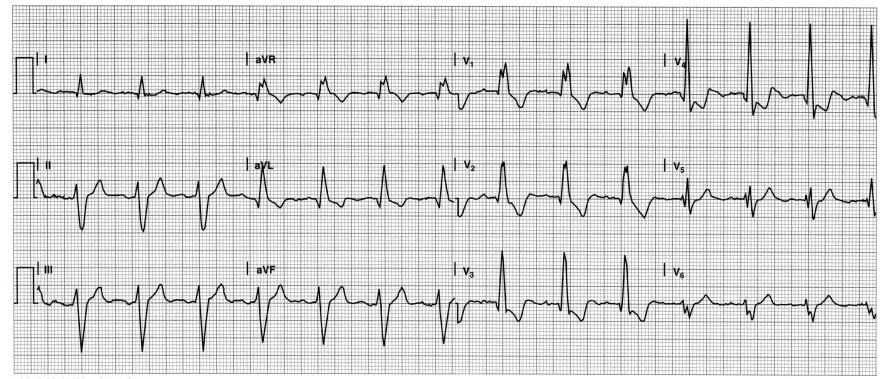

x1.0 0.05-150Hz 25mm/sec

Rate and rhythm? _____ Pathologic Q waves? _____

STE? _____ ST depression? _____ T-wave changes? _____

Reciprocal changes? _____ STE variant present? _____ Axis? _____

Interpretation: _____

Inferior: II, III, aVF | Septum: V$_1$, V$_2$ | Anterior: V$_3$, V$_4$ | **Lateral: I, aVL, V$_5$, V$_6$**

Fig. **5.39**

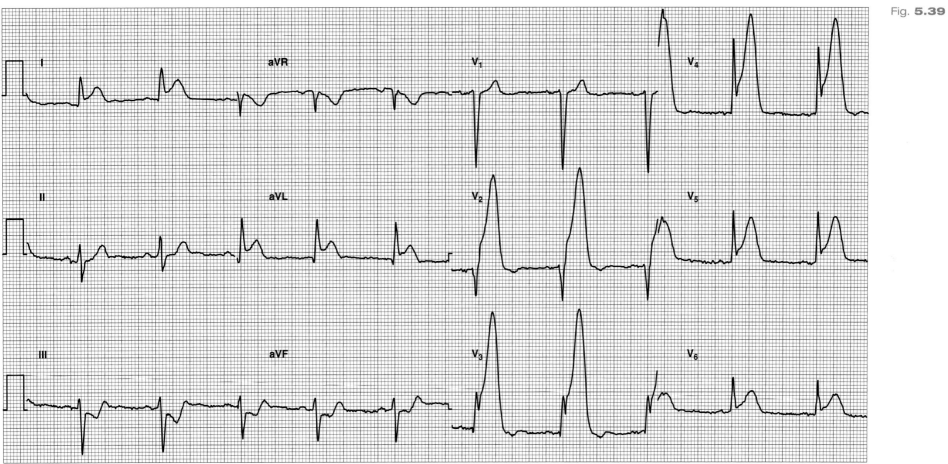

Rate and rhythm? _____ Pathologic Q waves? _____

STE? _____ ST depression? _____ T-wave changes? _____

Reciprocal changes? _____ STE variant present? _____ Axis? _____

Interpretation: _____

Inferior: II, III, aVF | Septum: V₁, V₂ | Anterior: V₃, V₄ | **Lateral: I, aVL, V₅, V₆**

Fig. **5.40**

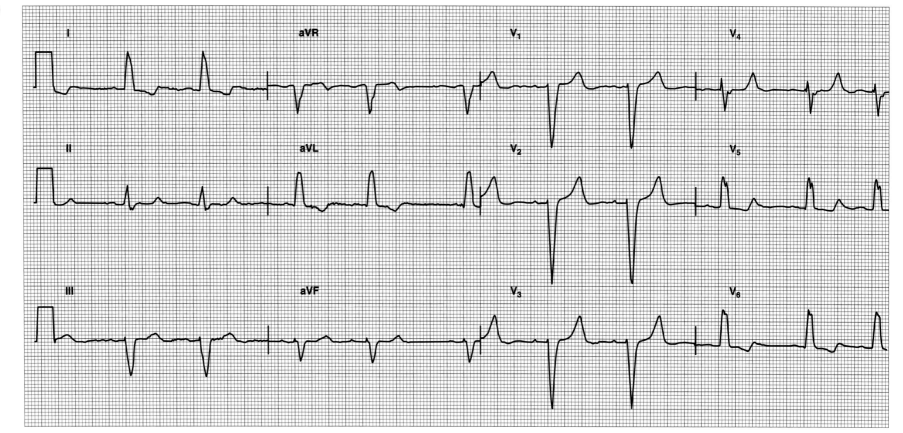

Rate and rhythm? _____ Pathologic Q waves? _____

STE? _____ ST depression? _____ T-wave changes? _____

Reciprocal changes? _____ STE variant present? _____ Axis? _____

Interpretation: _____

Inferior: II, III, aVF | **Septum: V₁, V₂** | **Anterior: V₃, V₄** | **Lateral: I, aVL, V₅, V₆**

Fig. **5.41**

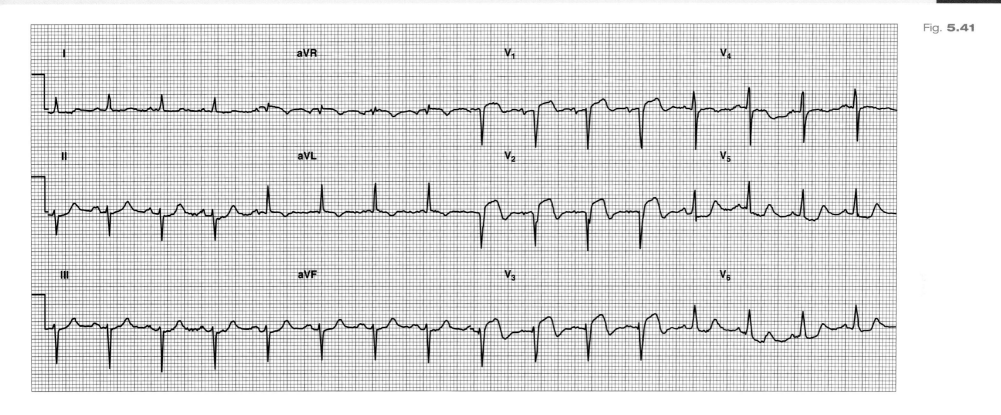

Rate and rhythm? _____ Pathologic Q waves? _____

STE? _____ ST depression? _____ T-wave changes? _____

Reciprocal changes? _____ STE variant present? _____ Axis? _____

Interpretation: _____

Inferior: II, III, aVF | Septum: V₁, V₂ | Anterior: V₃, V₄ | Lateral: I, aVL, V₅, V₆

Fig. **5.42**

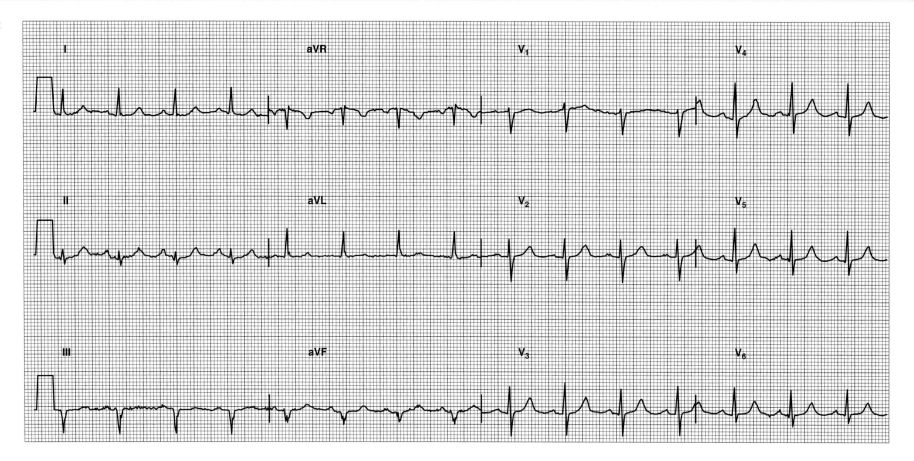

Rate and rhythm? _____ Pathologic Q waves? _____

STE? _____ ST depression? _____ T-wave changes? _____

Reciprocal changes? _____ STE variant present? _____ Axis? _____

Interpretation: _____

Inferior: II, III, aVF | Septum: V₁, V₂ | Anterior: V₃, V₄ | **Lateral: I, aVL, V₅, V₆**

Fig. **5.43**

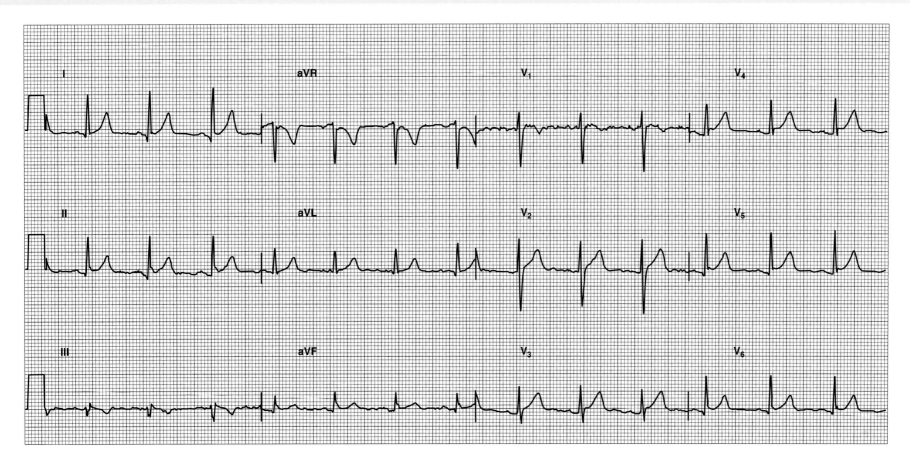

Rate and rhythm? _____ Pathologic Q waves? _____

STE? _____ ST depression? _____ T-wave changes? _____

Reciprocal changes? _____ STE variant present? _____ Axis? _____

Interpretation: _____

Inferior: II, III, aVF | Septum: V₁, V₂ | Anterior: V₃, V₄ | Lateral: I, aVL, V₅, V₆

Fig. **5.44**

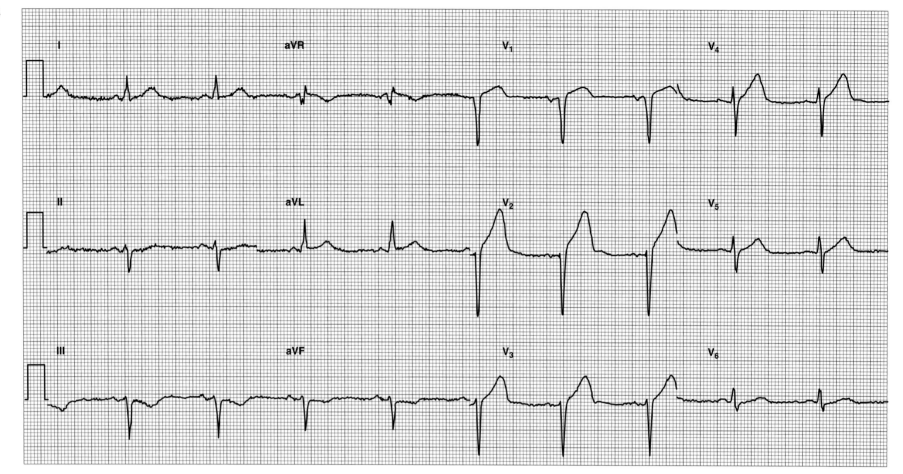

Rate and rhythm? _____ Pathologic Q waves? _____

STE? _____ ST depression? _____ T-wave changes? _____

Reciprocal changes? _____ STE variant present? _____ Axis? _____

Interpretation: _____

Inferior: II, III, aVF | Septum: V₁, V₂ | Anterior: V₃, V₄ | Lateral: I, aVL, V₅, V₆

Fig. **5.45**

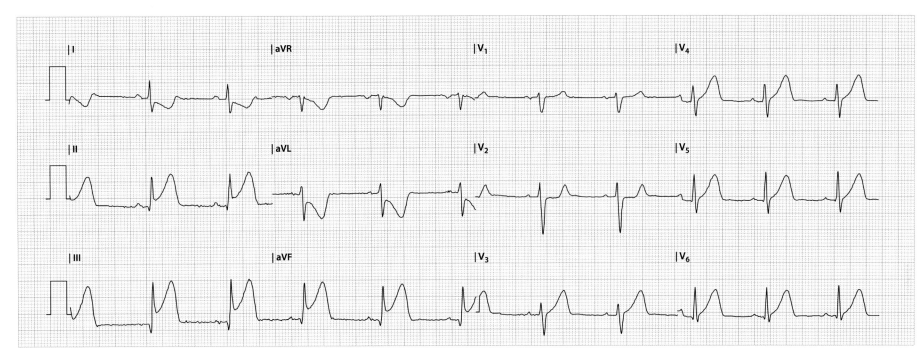

Rate and rhythm? _____ Pathologic Q waves? _____

STE? _____ ST depression? _____ T-wave changes? _____

Reciprocal changes? _____ STE variant present? _____ Axis? _____

Interpretation: _____

Inferior: II, III, aVF | **Septum: V₁, V₂** | Anterior: V₃, V₄ | **Lateral: I, aVL, V₅, V₆**

Fig. **5.46**

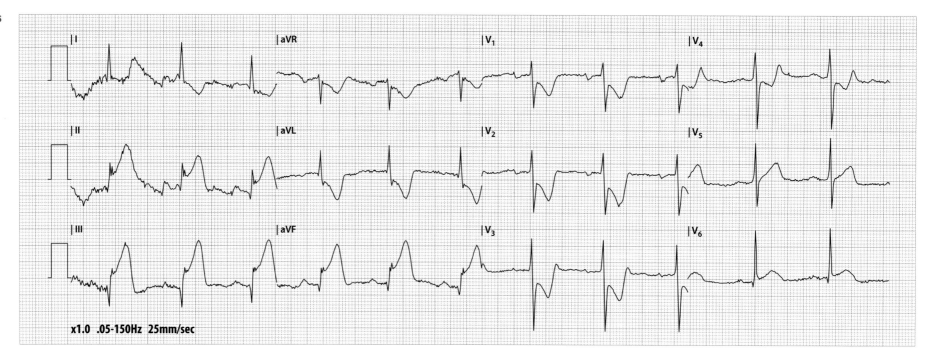

Rate and rhythm? _____ Pathologic Q waves? _____

STE? _____ ST depression? _____ T-wave changes? _____

Reciprocal changes? _____ STE variant present? _____ Axis? _____

Interpretation: _____

Inferior: II, III, aVF | **Septum: V$_1$, V$_2$** | **Anterior: V$_3$, V$_4$** | **Lateral: I, aVL, V$_5$, V$_6$**

Fig. **5.47**

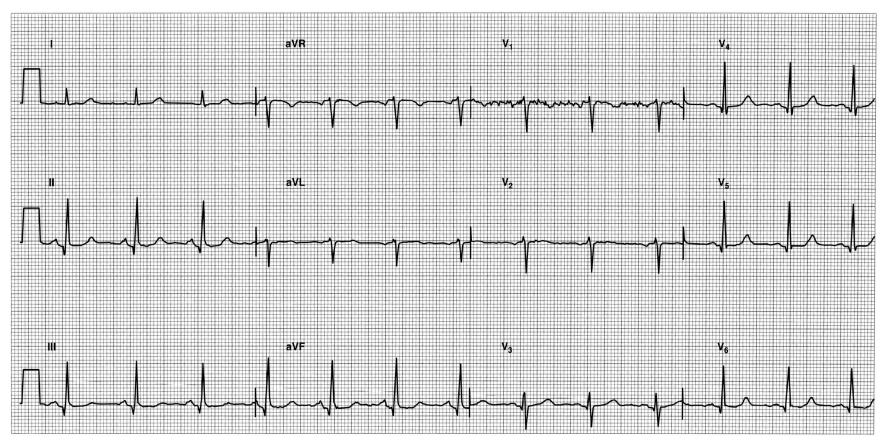

Rate and rhythm? _____ Pathologic Q waves? _____

STE? _____ ST depression? _____ T-wave changes? _____

Reciprocal changes? _____ STE variant present? _____ Axis? _____

Interpretation: _____

Inferior: II, III, aVF | Septum: V₁, V₂ | Anterior: V₃, V₄ | Lateral: I, aVL, V₅, V₆

Fig. **5.48**

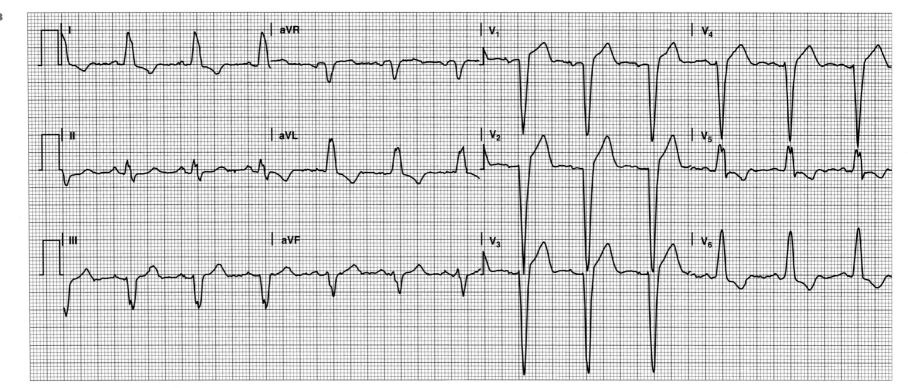

Rate and rhythm? _____ Pathologic Q waves? _____

STE? _____ ST depression? _____ T-wave changes? _____

Reciprocal changes? _____ STE variant present? _____ Axis? _____

Interpretation: _____

Inferior: II, III, aVF | Septum: V$_1$, V$_2$ | Anterior: V$_3$, V$_4$ | Lateral: I, aVL, V$_5$, V$_6$

Fig. **5.49**

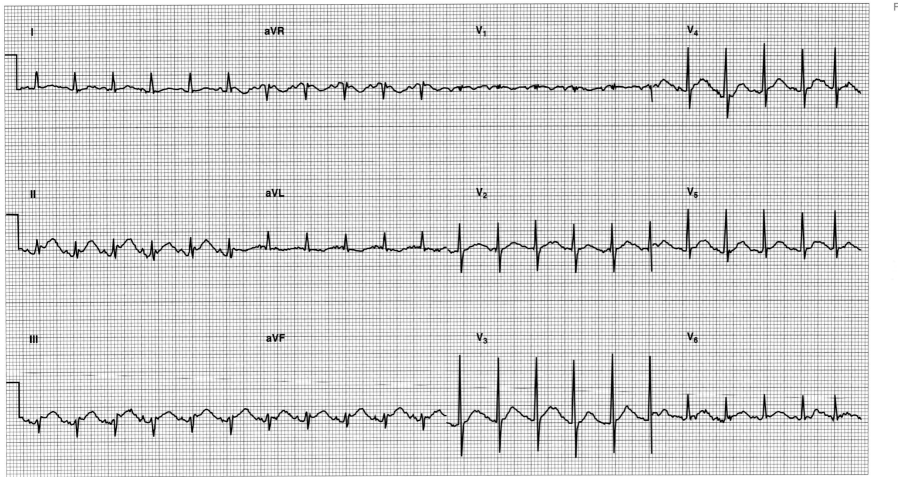

Rate and rhythm? _____ Pathologic Q waves? _____

STE? _____ ST depression? _____ T-wave changes? _____

Reciprocal changes? _____ STE variant present? _____ Axis? _____

Interpretation: _____

Inferior: II, III, aVF | Septum: V$_1$, V$_2$ | Anterior: V$_3$, V$_4$ | Lateral: I, aVL, V$_5$, V$_6$

Fig. **5.50**

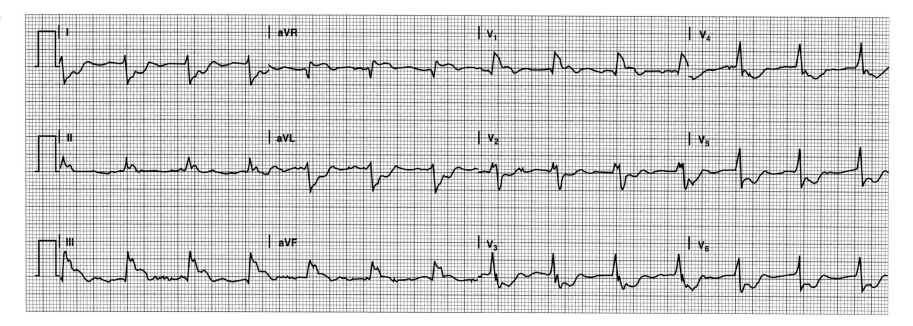

Rate and rhythm? _____ Pathologic Q waves? _____

STE? _____ ST depression? _____ T-wave changes? _____

Reciprocal changes? _____ STE variant present? _____ Axis? _____

Interpretation: _____

Inferior: II, III, aVF | Septum: V₁, V₂ | Anterior: V₃, V₄ | Lateral: I, aVL, V₅, V₆

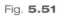

Fig. **5.51**

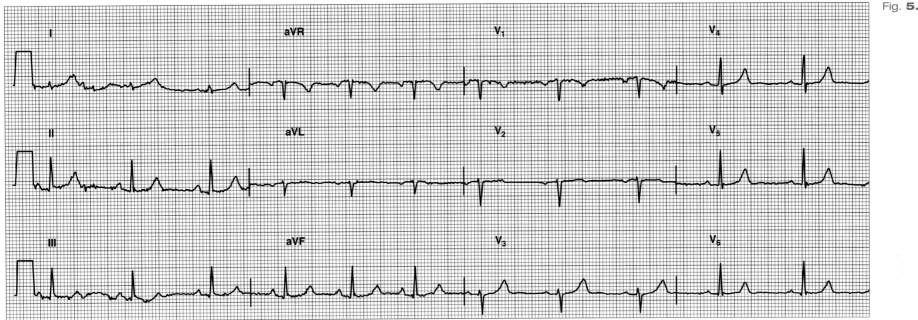

Rate and rhythm? _____ Pathologic Q waves? _____

STE? _____ ST depression? _____ T-wave changes? _____

Reciprocal changes? _____ STE variant present? _____ Axis? _____

Interpretation: _____

Inferior: II, III, aVF | Septum: V₁, V₂ | Anterior: V₃, V₄ | Lateral: I, aVL, V₅, V₆

Fig. **5.52**

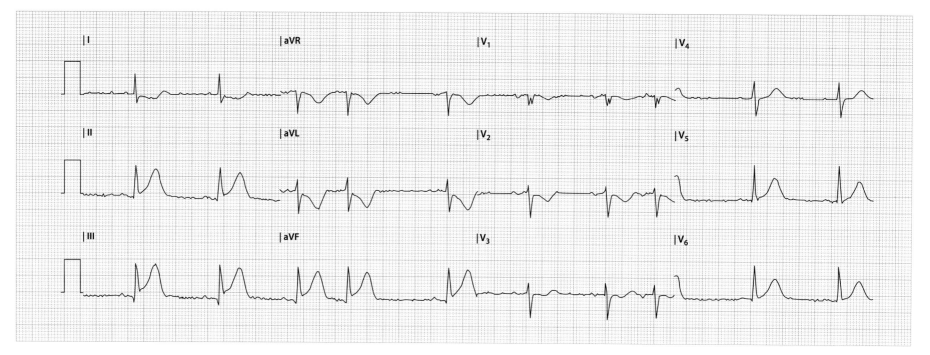

Rate and rhythm? _____ Pathologic Q waves? _____

STE? _____ ST depression? _____ T-wave changes? _____

Reciprocal changes? _____ STE variant present? _____ Axis? _____

Interpretation: _____

Inferior: II, III, aVF | Septum: V₁, V₂ | Anterior: V₃, V₄ | Lateral: I, aVL, V₅, V₆

Fig. **5.53**

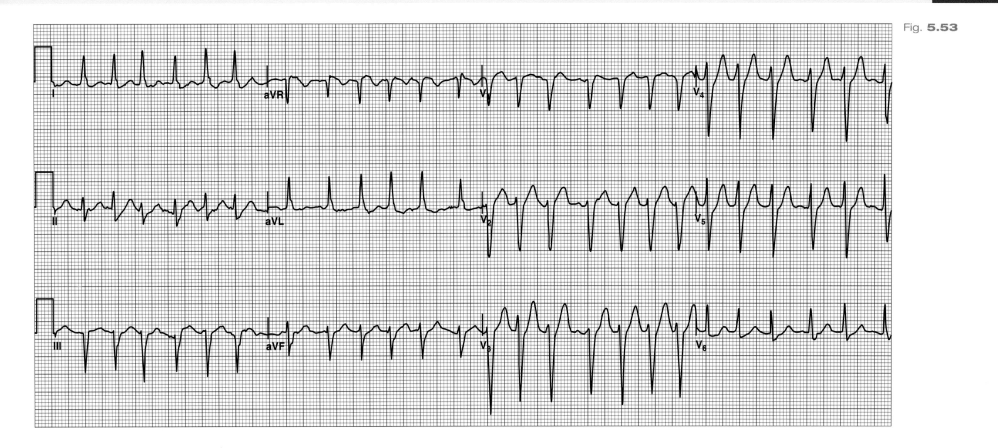

Rate and rhythm? _____ Pathologic Q waves? _____

STE? _____ ST depression? _____ T-wave changes? _____

Reciprocal changes? _____ STE variant present? _____ Axis? _____

Interpretation: _____

Inferior: II, III, aVF | Septum: V$_1$, V$_2$ | Anterior: V$_3$, V$_4$ | Lateral: I, aVL, V$_5$, V$_6$

Fig. **5.54**

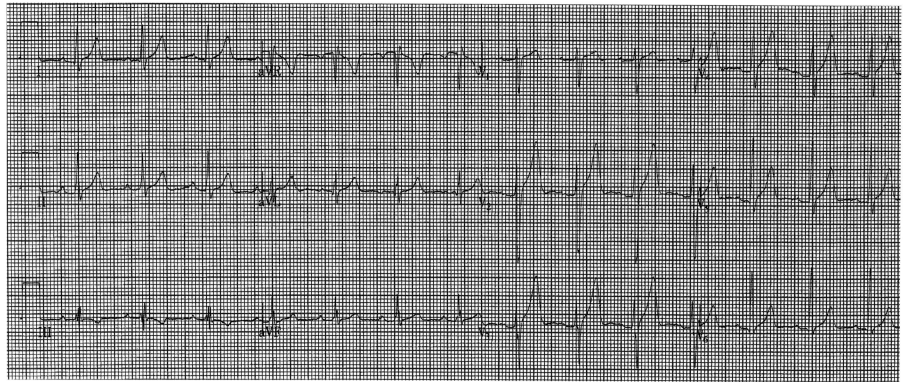

Rate and rhythm? _____ Pathologic Q waves? _____

STE? _____ ST depression? _____ T-wave changes? _____

Reciprocal changes? _____ STE variant present? _____ Axis? _____

Interpretation: _____

Inferior: II, III, aVF | Septum: V₁, V₂ | Anterior: V₃, V₄ | **Lateral: I, aVL, V₅, V₆**

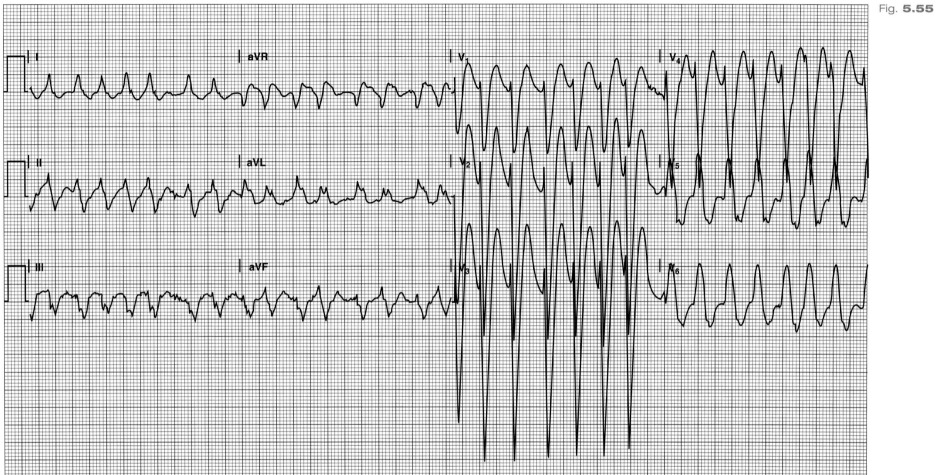

Fig. **5.55**

x1.0 0.05-150Hz 25mm/sec

Rate and rhythm? _____ Pathologic Q waves? _____

STE? _____ ST depression? _____ T-wave changes? _____

Reciprocal changes? _____ STE variant present? _____ Axis? _____

Interpretation: _____

Inferior: II, III, aVF | **Septum: V$_1$, V$_2$** | **Anterior: V$_3$, V$_4$** | **Lateral: I, aVL, V$_5$, V$_6$**

Fig. **5.56**

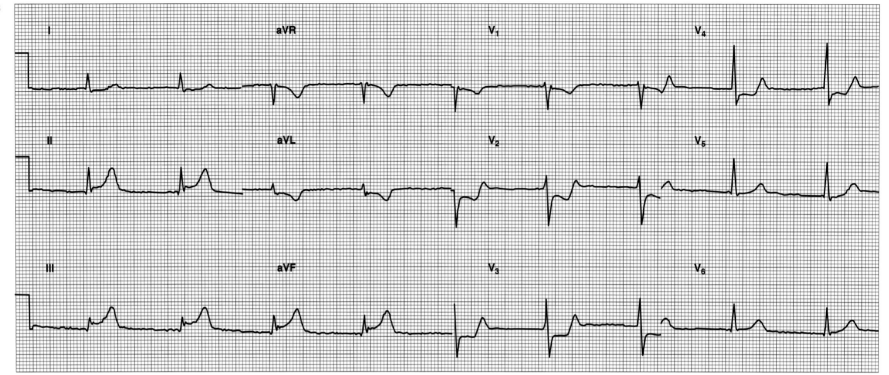

Rate and rhythm? _____ Pathologic Q waves? _____

STE? _____ ST depression? _____ T-wave changes? _____

Reciprocal changes? _____ STE variant present? _____ Axis? _____

Interpretation: _____

Inferior: II, III, aVF | Septum: V₁, V₂ | Anterior: V₃, V₄ | Lateral: I, aVL, V₅, V₆

Fig. **5.57**

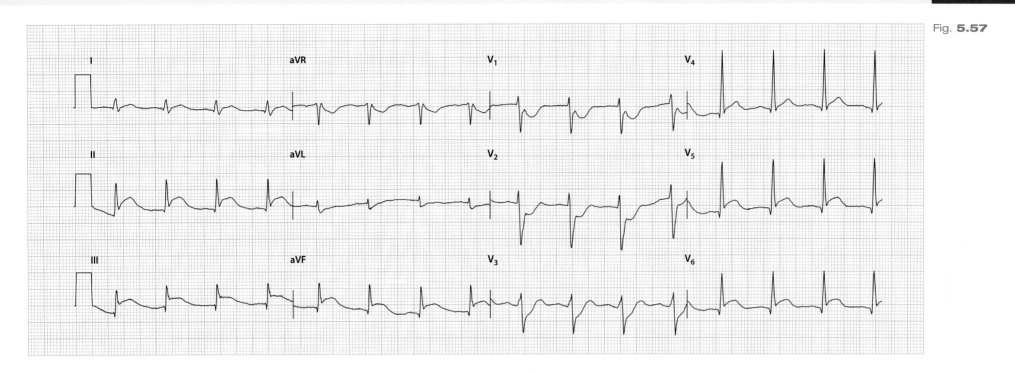

Rate and rhythm? _____ Pathologic Q waves? _____

STE? _____ ST depression? _____ T-wave changes? _____

Reciprocal changes? _____ STE variant present? _____ Axis? _____

Interpretation: _____

Inferior: II, III, aVF | **Septum: V₁, V₂** | Anterior: V₃, V₄ | **Lateral: I, aVL, V₅, V₆**

Fig. **5.58**

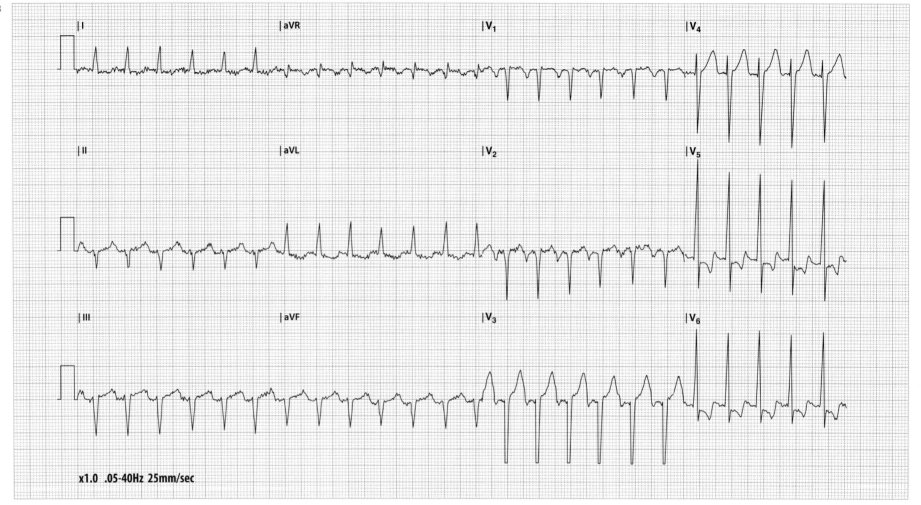

x1.0 .05-40Hz 25mm/sec

Rate and rhythm? _____ Pathologic Q waves? _____

STE? _____ ST depression? _____ T-wave changes? _____

Reciprocal changes? _____ STE variant present? _____ Axis? _____

Interpretation: _____

Inferior: II, III, aVF | Septum: V₁, V₂ | Anterior: V₃, V₄ | Lateral: I, aVL, V₅, V₆

Fig. **5.59**

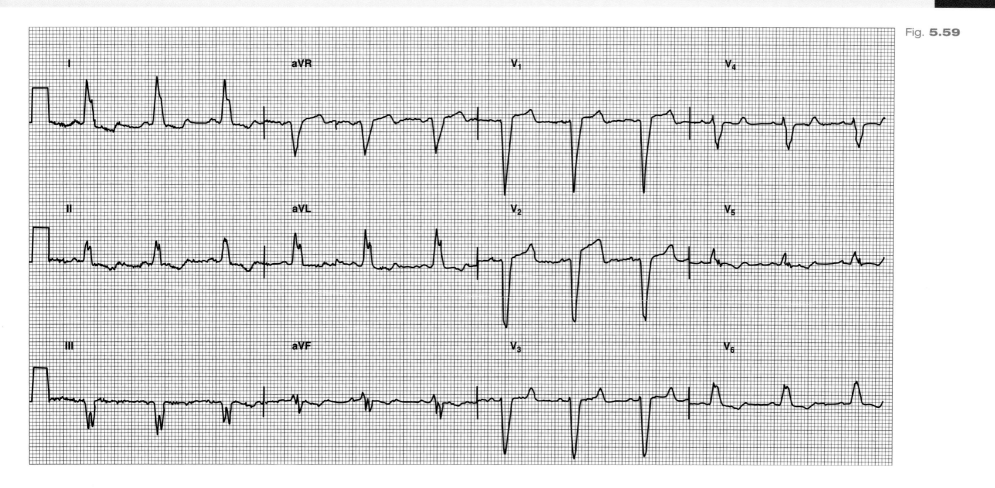

Rate and rhythm? _____ Pathologic Q waves? _____

STE? _____ ST depression? _____ T-wave changes? _____

Reciprocal changes? _____ STE variant present? _____ Axis? _____

Interpretation: _____

Inferior: II, III, aVF | Septum: V₁, V₂ | Anterior: V₃, V₄ | Lateral: I, aVL, V₅, V₆

Fig. **5.60**

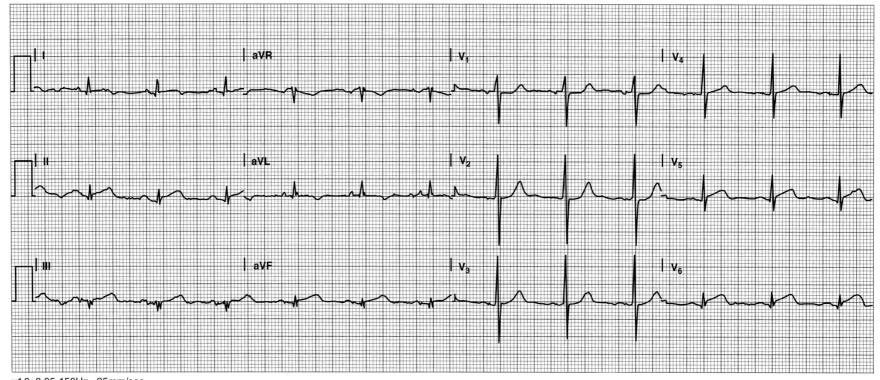

x1.0 0.05-150Hz   25mm/sec

Rate and rhythm? _____ Pathologic Q waves? _____

STE? _____ ST depression? _____ T-wave changes? _____

Reciprocal changes? _____ STE variant present? _____ Axis? _____

Interpretation: _____

Inferior: II, III, aVF | Septum: V$_1$, V$_2$ | Anterior: V$_3$, V$_4$ | Lateral: I, aVL, V$_5$, V$_6$

Fig. **5.61**

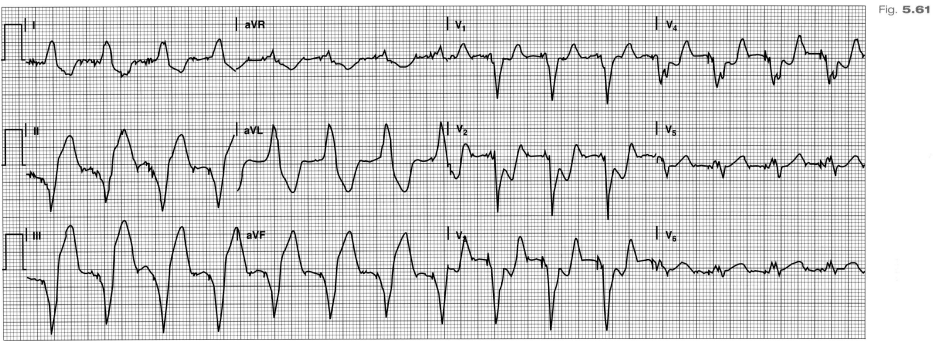

x1.0 0.05-150Hz   25mm/sec

Rate and rhythm? _____ Pathologic Q waves? _____

STE? _____ ST depression? _____ T-wave changes? _____

Reciprocal changes? _____ STE variant present? _____ Axis? _____

Interpretation: _____

Inferior: II, III, aVF | **Septum: V$_1$, V$_2$** | **Anterior: V$_3$, V$_4$** | **Lateral: I, aVL, V$_5$, V$_6$**

Fig. **5.62**

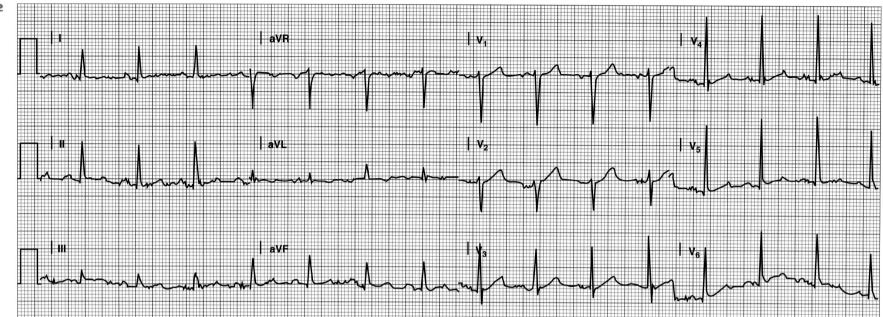

Rate and rhythm? _____ Pathologic Q waves? _____

STE? _____ ST depression? _____ T-wave changes? _____

Reciprocal changes? _____ STE variant present? _____ Axis? _____

Interpretation: _____

Inferior: II, III, aVF | Septum: V₁, V₂ | Anterior: V₃, V₄ | Lateral: I, aVL, V₅, V₆

Fig. **5.63**

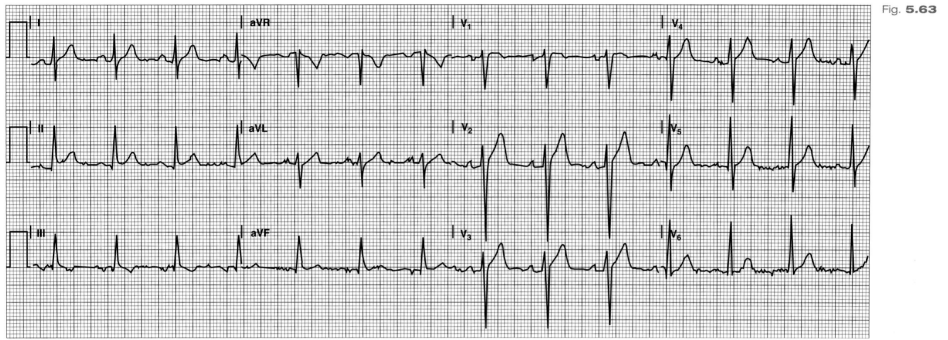

Rate and rhythm? _____ Pathologic Q waves? _____

STE? _____ ST depression? _____ T-wave changes? _____

Reciprocal changes? _____ STE variant present? _____ Axis? _____

Interpretation: _____

Inferior: II, III, aVF | Septum: V₁, V₂ | Anterior: V₃, V₄ | Lateral: I, aVL, V₅, V₆

Fig. **5.64**

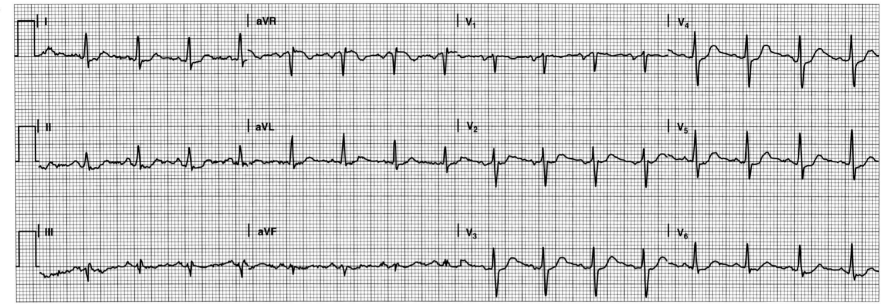

Rate and rhythm? _____   Pathologic Q waves? _____

STE? _____ ST depression? _____ T-wave changes? _____

Reciprocal changes? _____ STE variant present? _____ Axis? _____

Interpretation: _____

Inferior: II, III, aVF | Septum: V$_1$, V$_2$ | Anterior: V$_3$, V$_4$ | Lateral: I, aVL, V$_5$, V$_6$

Fig. 5.65

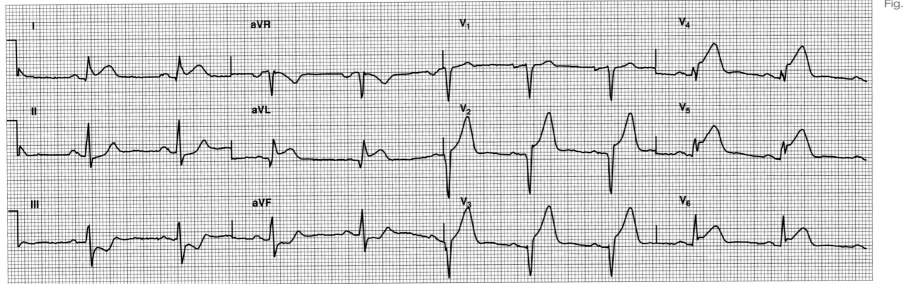

Rate and rhythm? _____ Pathologic Q waves? _____

STE? _____ ST depression? _____ T-wave changes? _____

Reciprocal changes? _____ STE variant present? _____ Axis? _____

Interpretation: _____

Inferior: II, III, aVF | Septum: V₁, V₂ | Anterior: V₃, V₄ | Lateral: I, aVL, V₅, V₆

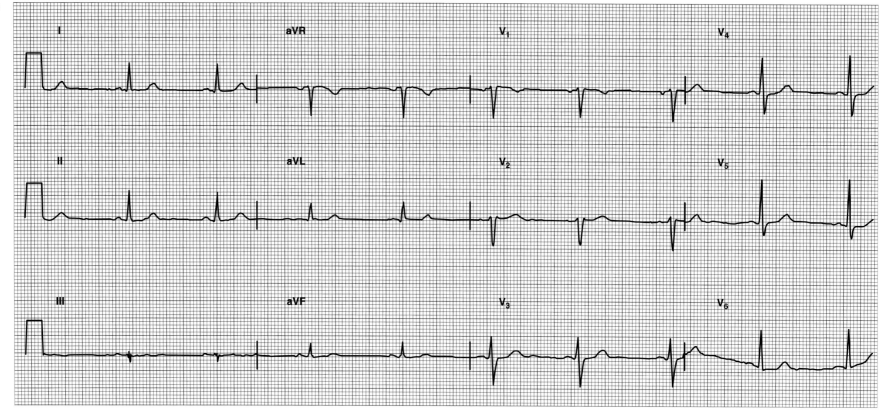

Rate and rhythm? _____ Pathologic Q waves? _____

STE? _____ ST depression? _____ T-wave changes? _____

Reciprocal changes? _____ STE variant present? _____ Axis? _____

Interpretation: _____

Inferior: II, III, aVF | Septum: V₁, V₂ | Anterior: V₃, V₄ | Lateral: I, aVL, V₅, V₆

Fig. **5.67**

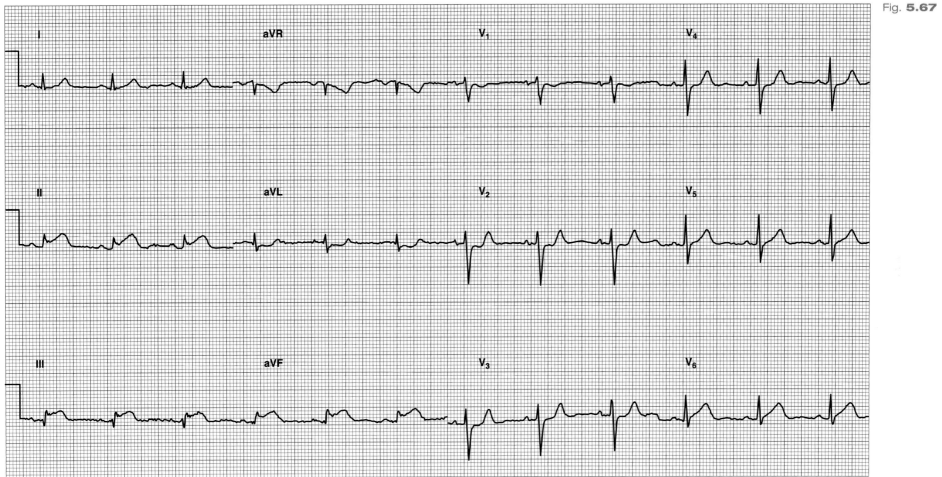

Rate and rhythm? _____ Pathologic Q waves? _____

STE? _____ ST depression? _____ T-wave changes? _____

Reciprocal changes? _____ STE variant present? _____ Axis? _____

Interpretation: _____

Inferior: II, III, aVF | **Septum: V₁, V₂** | **Anterior: V₃, V₄** | **Lateral: I, aVL, V₅, V₆**

Fig. **5.68**

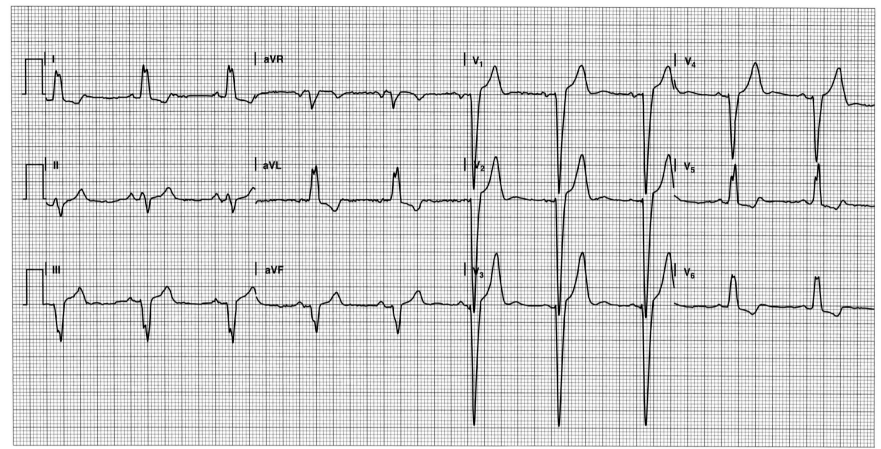

x1.0 0.05-150Hz 25mm/sec

Rate and rhythm? _____ Pathologic Q waves? _____

STE? _____ ST depression? _____ T-wave changes? _____

Reciprocal changes? _____ STE variant present? _____ Axis? _____

Interpretation: _____

Inferior: II, III, aVF | Septum: V₁, V₂ | Anterior: V₃, V₄ | Lateral: I, aVL, V₅, V₆

Fig. **5.69**

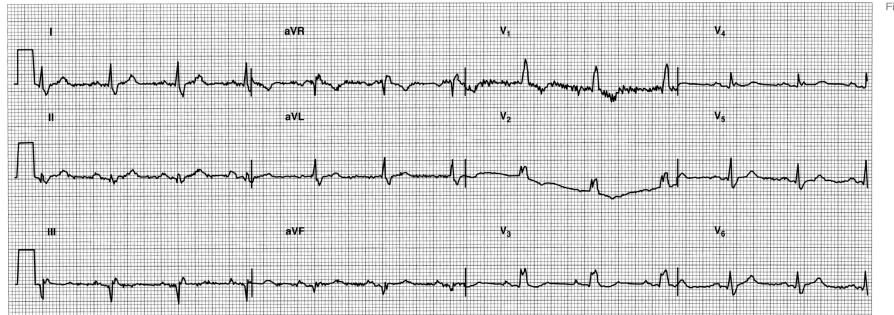

Rate and rhythm? _____ Pathologic Q waves? _____

STE? _____ ST depression? _____ T-wave changes? _____

Reciprocal changes? _____ STE variant present? _____ Axis? _____

Interpretation: _____

Inferior: II, III, aVF | **Septum: V₁, V₂** | **Anterior: V₃, V₄** | **Lateral: I, aVL, V₅, V₆**

Fig. **5.70**

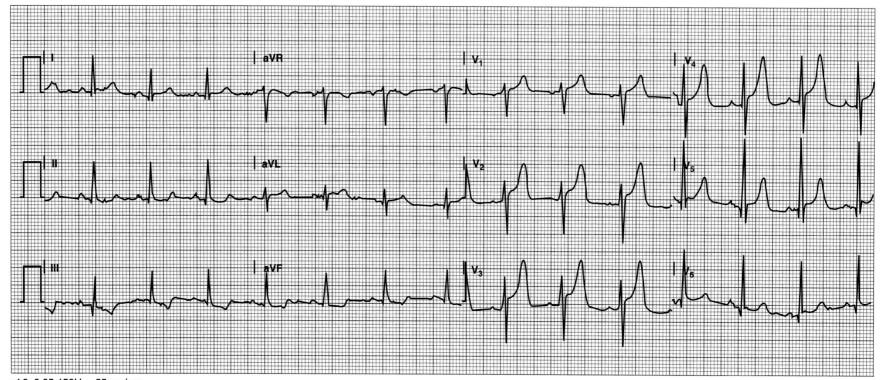

x1.0 0.05-150Hz 25mm/sec

Rate and rhythm? _____ Pathologic Q waves? _____

STE? _____ ST depression? _____ T-wave changes? _____

Reciprocal changes? _____ STE variant present? _____ Axis? _____

Interpretation: _____

Inferior: II, III, aVF | Septum: V_1, V_2 | Anterior: V_3, V_4 | Lateral: I, aVL, V_5, V_6

Fig. **5.71**

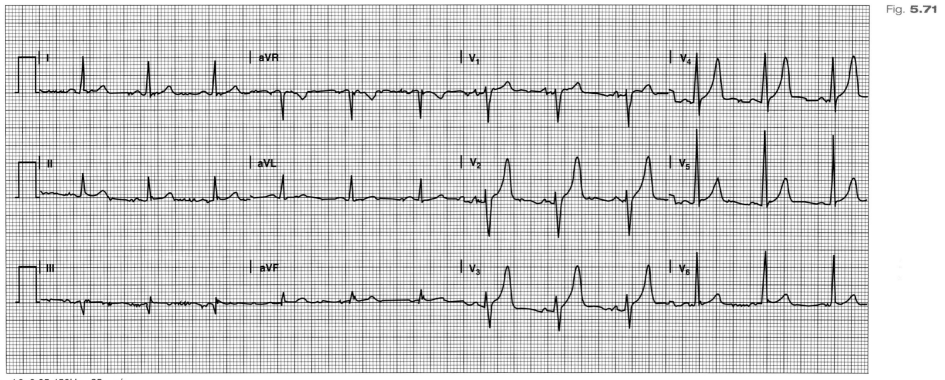

x1.0 0.05-150Hz   25mm/sec

Rate and rhythm? _____ Pathologic Q waves? _____

STE? _____ ST depression? _____ T-wave changes? _____

Reciprocal changes? _____ STE variant present? _____ Axis? _____

Interpretation: _____

Inferior: II, III, aVF | Septum: V$_1$, V$_2$ | Anterior: V$_3$, V$_4$ | Lateral: I, aVL, V$_5$, V$_6$

Fig. **5.72**

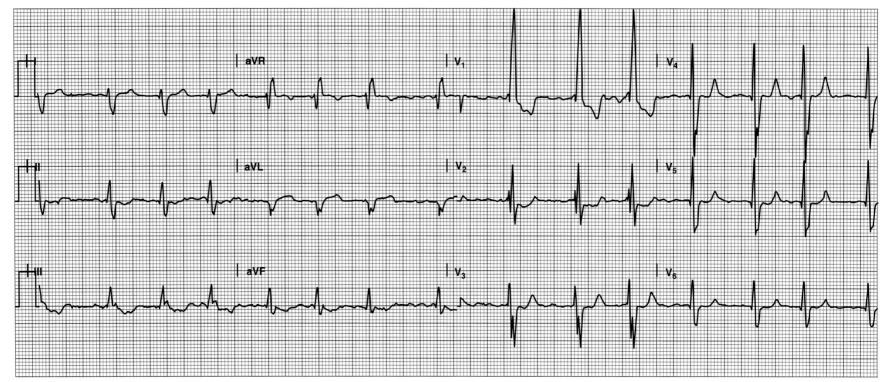

x1.0 0.05-150Hz 25mm/sec

Rate and rhythm? _____ Pathologic Q waves? _____

STE? _____ ST depression? _____ T-wave changes? _____

Reciprocal changes? _____ STE variant present? _____ Axis? _____

Interpretation: _____

Inferior: II, III, aVF | Septum: V$_1$, V$_2$ | Anterior: V$_3$, V$_4$ | Lateral: I, aVL, V$_5$, V$_6$

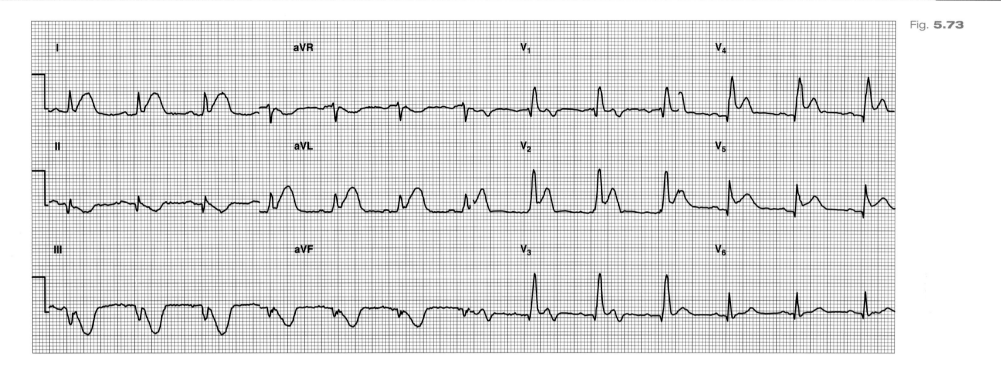

Fig. **5.73**

Rate and rhythm? _____ Pathologic Q waves? _____

STE? _____ ST depression? _____ T-wave changes? _____

Reciprocal changes? _____ STE variant present? _____ Axis? _____

Interpretation: _____

Inferior: II, III, aVF | Septum: V₁, V₂ | Anterior: V₃, V₄ | Lateral: I, aVL, V₅, V₆

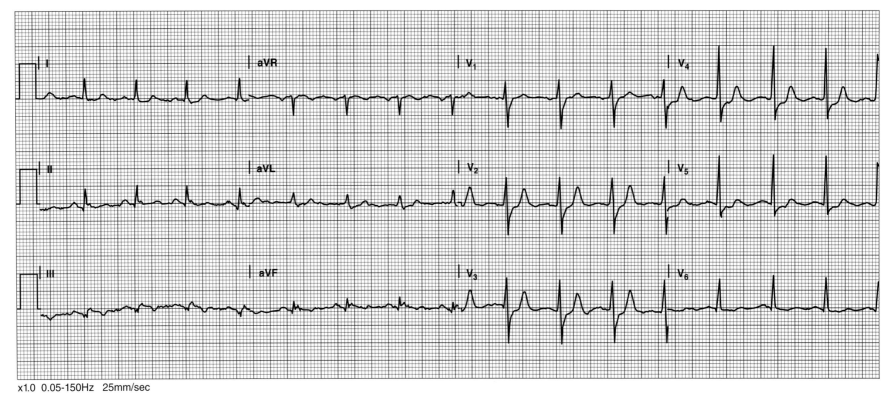

x1.0 0.05-150Hz 25mm/sec

Rate and rhythm? _____ Pathologic Q waves? _____

STE? _____ ST depression? _____ T-wave changes? _____

Reciprocal changes? _____ STE variant present? _____ Axis? _____

Interpretation: _____

Inferior: II, III, aVF | **Septum: V₁, V₂** | **Anterior: V₃, V₄** | **Lateral: I, aVL, V₅, V₆**

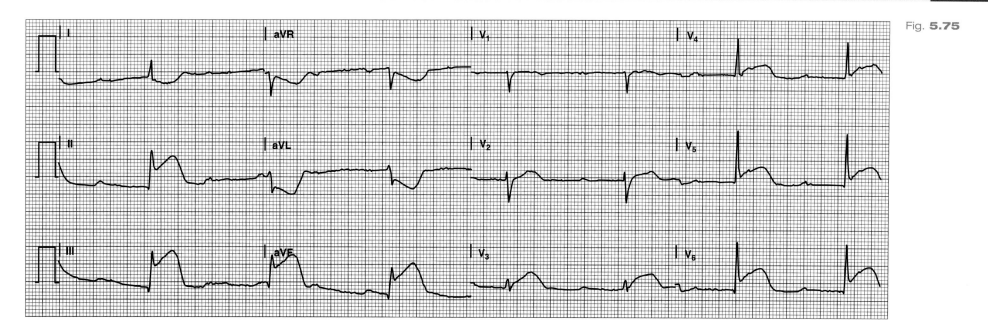

Fig. **5.75**

Rate and rhythm? _____ Pathologic Q waves? _____

STE? _____ ST depression? _____ T-wave changes? _____

Reciprocal changes? _____ STE variant present? _____ Axis? _____

Interpretation: _____

Inferior: II, III, aVF | Septum: V₁, V₂ | Anterior: V₃, V₄ | Lateral: I, aVL, V₅, V₆

Fig. **5.76**

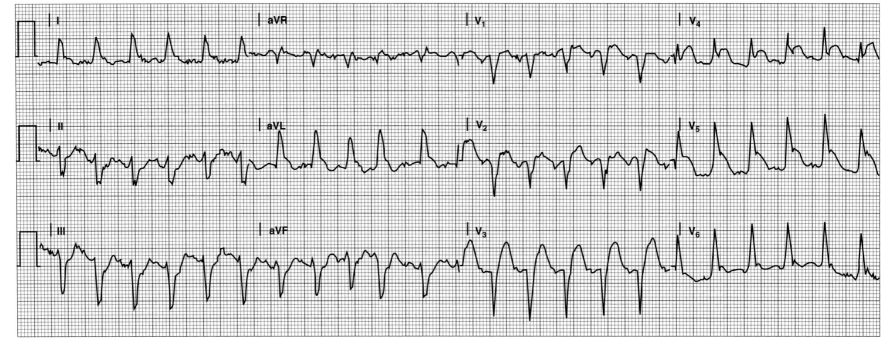

Rate and rhythm? _____   Pathologic Q waves? _____

STE? _____   ST depression? _____   T-wave changes? _____

Reciprocal changes? _____   STE variant present? _____   Axis? _____

Interpretation: _____

Inferior: II, III, aVF | Septum: V₁, V₂ | Anterior: V₃, V₄ | Lateral: I, aVL, V₅, V₆

Fig. **5.77**

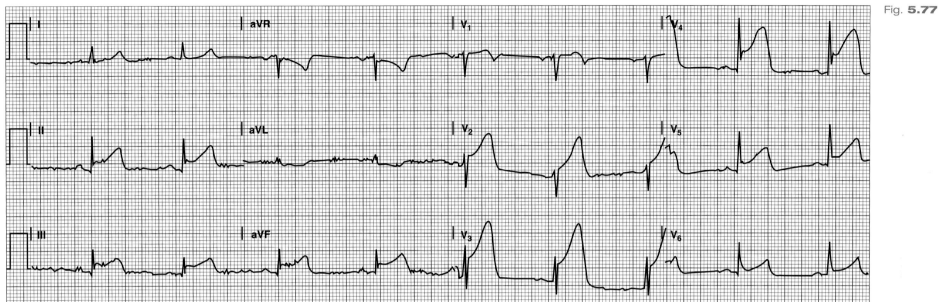

Rate and rhythm? _____ Pathologic Q waves? _____

STE? _____ ST depression? _____ T-wave changes? _____

Reciprocal changes? _____ STE variant present? _____ Axis? _____

Interpretation: _____

Inferior: II, III, aVF | **Septum: V₁, V₂** | **Anterior: V₃, V₄** | **Lateral: I, aVL, V₅, V₆**

Fig. **5.78**

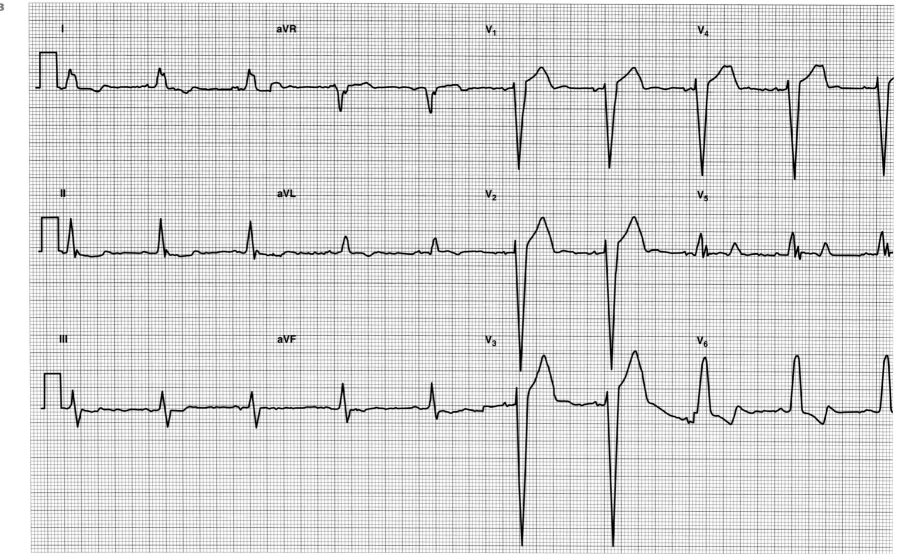

Rate and rhythm? _____ Pathologic Q waves? _____

STE? _____ ST depression? _____ T-wave changes? _____

Reciprocal changes? _____ STE variant present? _____ Axis? _____

Interpretation: _____

Inferior: II, III, aVF | **Septum: V₁, V₂** | **Anterior: V₃, V₄** | **Lateral: I, aVL, V₅, V₆**

Fig. **5.79**

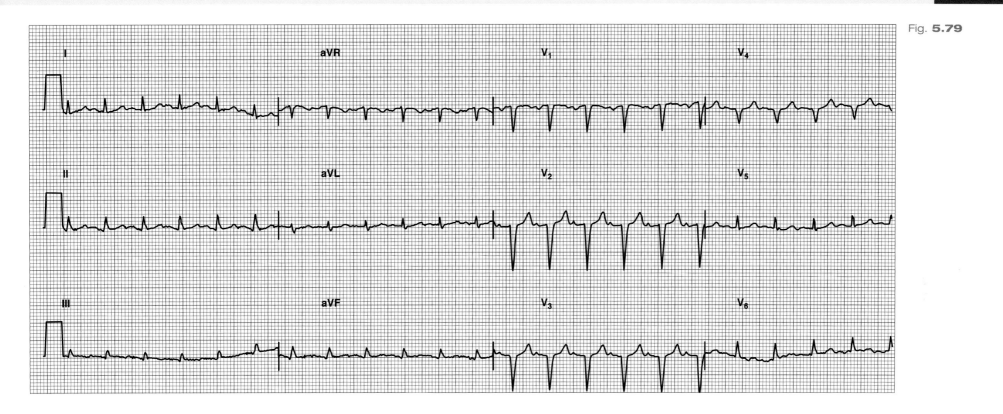

Rate and rhythm? _____ Pathologic Q waves? _____

STE? _____ ST depression? _____ T-wave changes? _____

Reciprocal changes? _____ STE variant present? _____ Axis? _____

Interpretation: _____

Inferior: II, III, aVF | **Septum: V$_1$, V$_2$** | **Anterior: V$_3$, V$_4$** | **Lateral: I, aVL, V$_5$, V$_6$**

Fig. 5.80

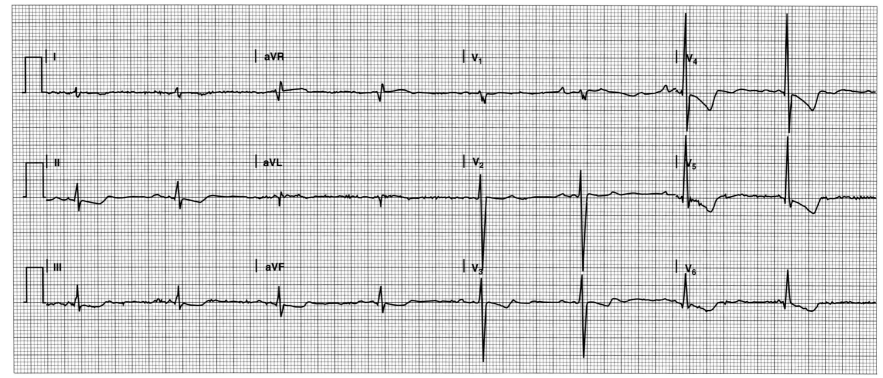

x1.0 0.05-150Hz 25mm/sec

Rate and rhythm? _____ Pathologic Q waves? _____

STE? _____ ST depression? _____ T-wave changes? _____

Reciprocal changes? _____ STE variant present? _____ Axis? _____

Interpretation: _____

Inferior: II, III, aVF | **Septum: V₁, V₂** | **Anterior: V₃, V₄** | **Lateral: I, aVL, V₅, V₆**

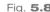

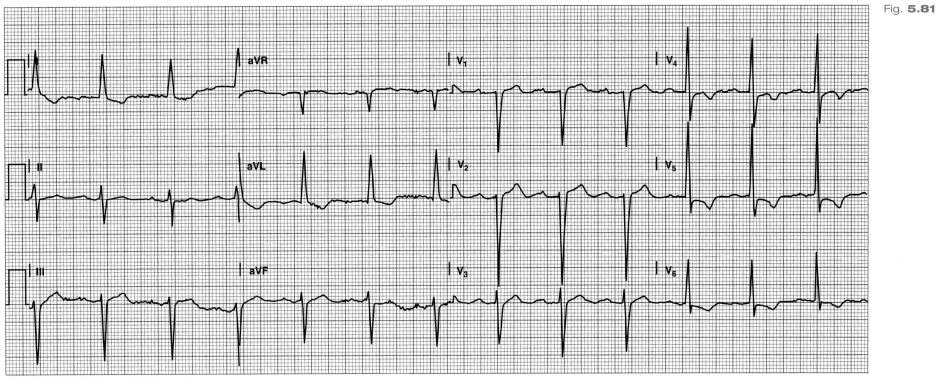

Fig. **5.81**

x1.0 0.05-150Hz   25mm/sec

Rate and rhythm? _____ Pathologic Q waves? _____

STE? _____ ST depression? _____ T-wave changes? _____

Reciprocal changes? _____ STE variant present? _____ Axis? _____

Interpretation: _____

Inferior: II, III, aVF | **Septum: V₁, V₂** | **Anterior: V₃, V₄** | **Lateral: I, aVL, V₅, V₆**

Fig. **5.82**

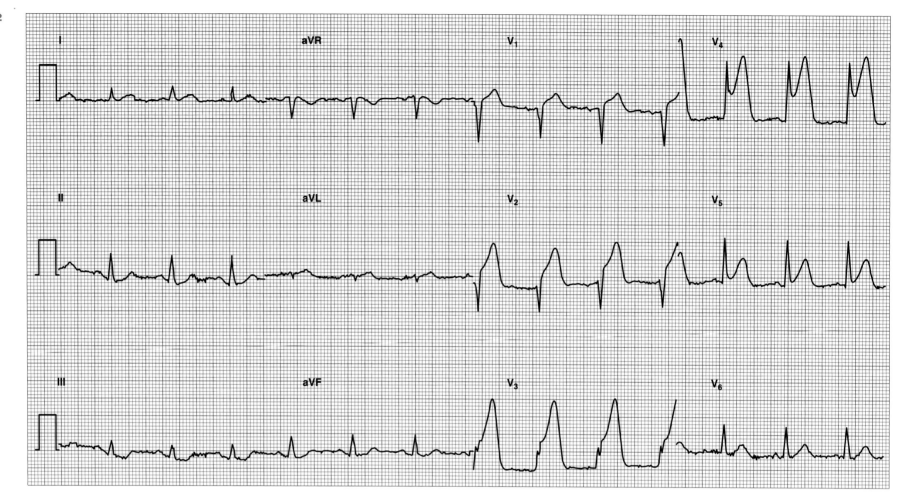

Rate and rhythm? _____ Pathologic Q waves? _____

STE? _____ ST depression? _____ T-wave changes? _____

Reciprocal changes? _____ STE variant present? _____ Axis? _____

Interpretation: _____

Inferior: II, III, aVF | Septum: V_1, V_2 | Anterior: V_3, V_4 | Lateral: I, aVL, V_5, V_6

Fig. 5.83

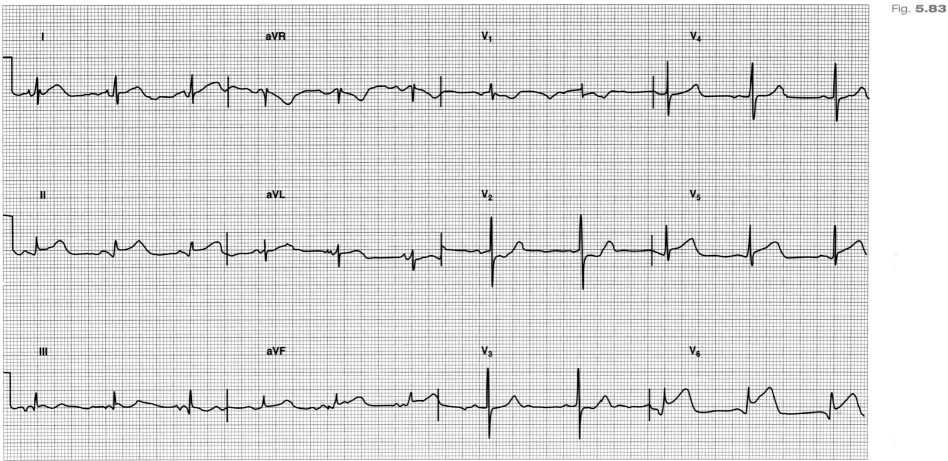

Rate and rhythm? _____ Pathologic Q waves? _____

STE? _____ ST depression? _____ T-wave changes? _____

Reciprocal changes? _____ STE variant present? _____ Axis? _____

Interpretation: _____

Inferior: II, III, aVF | Septum: V$_1$, V$_2$ | Anterior: V$_3$, V$_4$ | Lateral: I, aVL, V$_5$, V$_6$

Fig. **5.84**

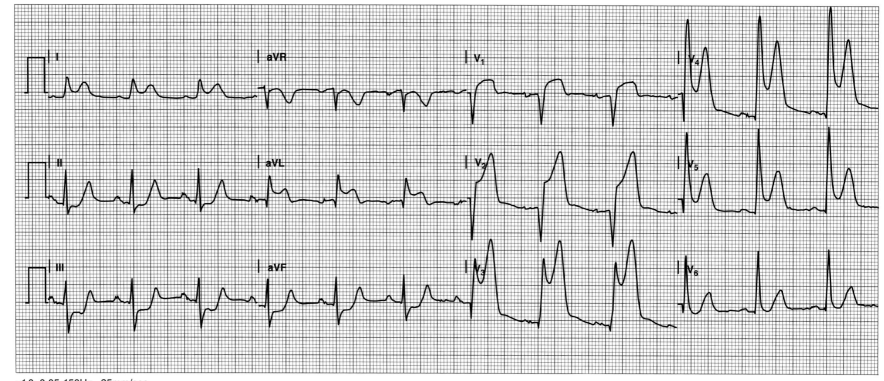

x1.0 0.05-150Hz   25mm/sec

Rate and rhythm? _____ Pathologic Q waves? _____

STE? _____ ST depression? _____ T-wave changes? _____

Reciprocal changes? _____ STE variant present? _____ Axis? _____

Interpretation: _____

Inferior: II, III, aVF | Septum: V$_1$, V$_2$ | Anterior: V$_3$, V$_4$ | Lateral: I, aVL, V$_5$, V$_6$

Fig. **5.85**

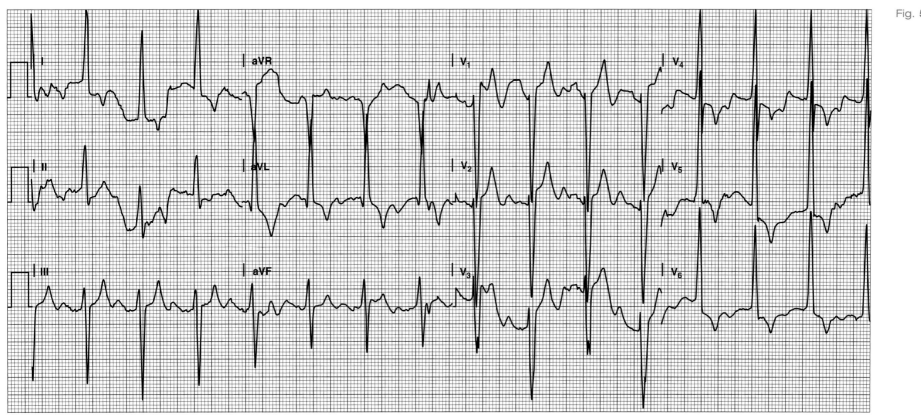

Rate and rhythm? _____ Pathologic Q waves? _____

STE? _____ ST depression? _____ T-wave changes? _____

Reciprocal changes? _____ STE variant present? _____ Axis? _____

Interpretation: _____

Inferior: II, III, aVF | Septum: V₁, V₂ | Anterior: V₃, V₄ | Lateral: I, aVL, V₅, V₆

Fig. **5.86**

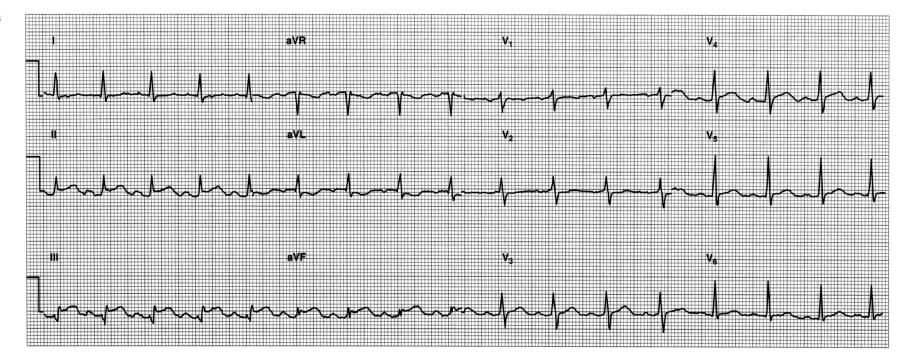

Rate and rhythm? _____ Pathologic Q waves? _____

STE? _____ ST depression? _____ T-wave changes? _____

Reciprocal changes? _____ STE variant present? _____ Axis? _____

Interpretation: _____

Inferior: II, III, aVF | **Septum: V₁, V₂** | **Anterior: V₃, V₄** | **Lateral: I, aVL, V₅, V₆**

Fig. **5.87**

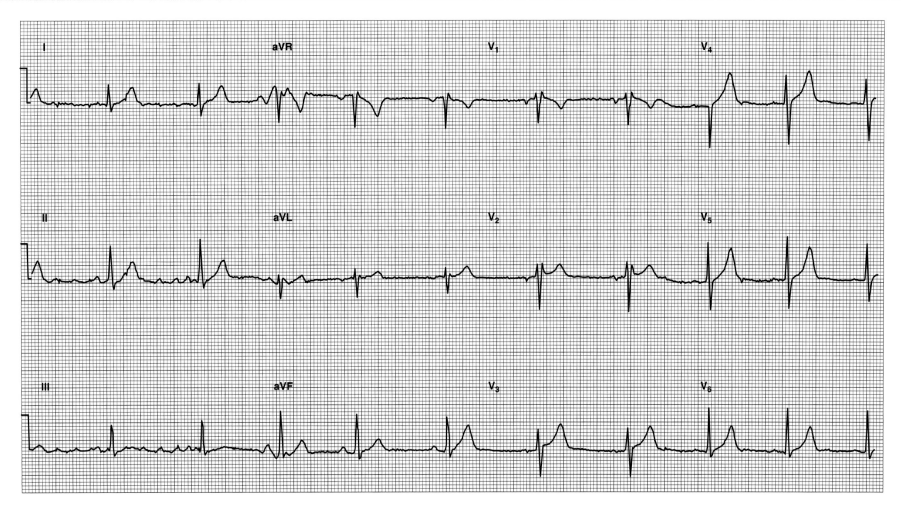

Rate and rhythm? _____ Pathologic Q waves? _____

STE? _____ ST depression? _____ T-wave changes? _____

Reciprocal changes? _____ STE variant present? _____ Axis? _____

Interpretation: _____

Inferior: II, III, aVF | Septum: V₁, V₂ | Anterior: V₃, V₄ | **Lateral: I, aVL, V₅, V₆**

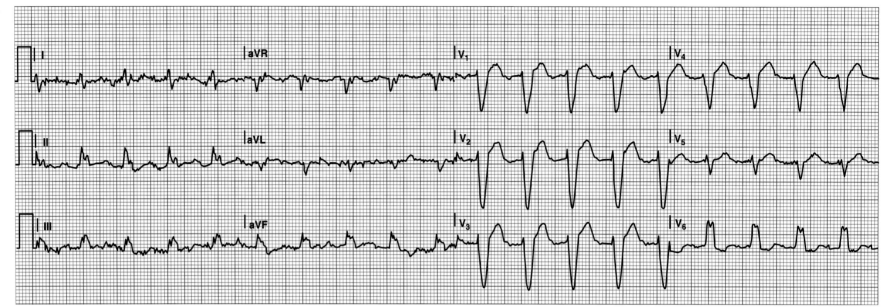

Fig. 5.88

Rate and rhythm? _____ Pathologic Q waves? _____

STE? _____ ST depression? _____ T-wave changes? _____

Reciprocal changes? _____ STE variant present? _____ Axis? _____

Interpretation: _____

Inferior: II, III, aVF | Septum: V₁, V₂ | Anterior: V₃, V₄ | Lateral: I, aVL, V₅, V₆

Fig. **5.89**

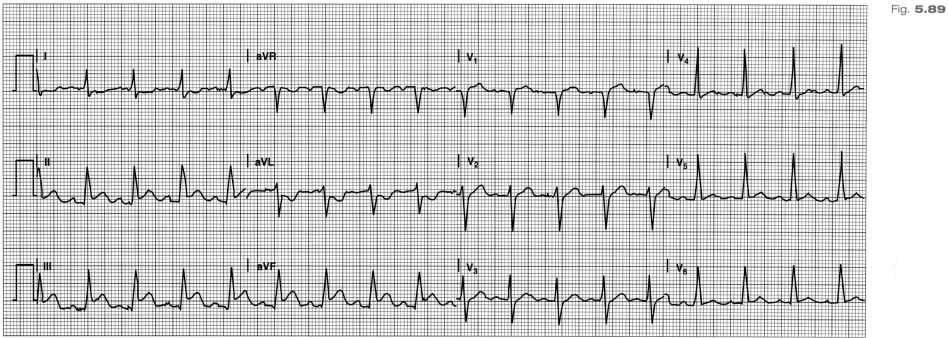

Rate and rhythm? _____ Pathologic Q waves? _____

STE? _____ ST depression? _____ T-wave changes? _____

Reciprocal changes? _____ STE variant present? _____ Axis? _____

Interpretation: _____

Inferior: II, III, aVF | Septum: V₁, V₂ | Anterior: V₃, V₄ | Lateral: I, aVL, V₅, V₆

Fig. **5.90**

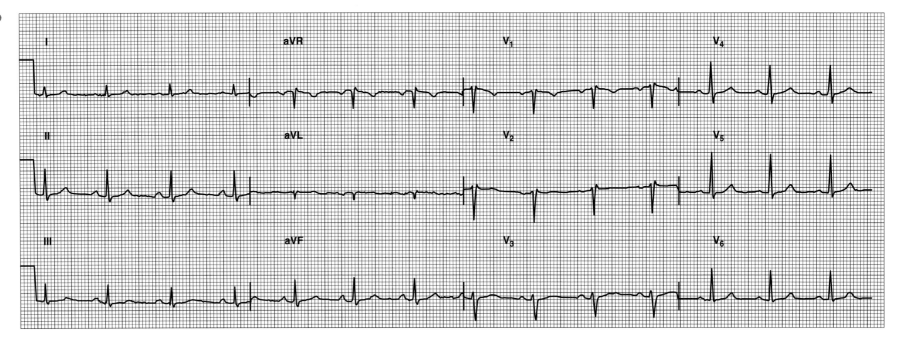

Rate and rhythm? _____ Pathologic Q waves? _____

STE? _____ ST depression? _____ T-wave changes? _____

Reciprocal changes? _____ STE variant present? _____ Axis? _____

Interpretation: _____

Inferior: II, III, aVF | Septum: V₁, V₂ | Anterior: V₃, V₄ | Lateral: I, aVL, V₅, V₆

Fig. **5.91**

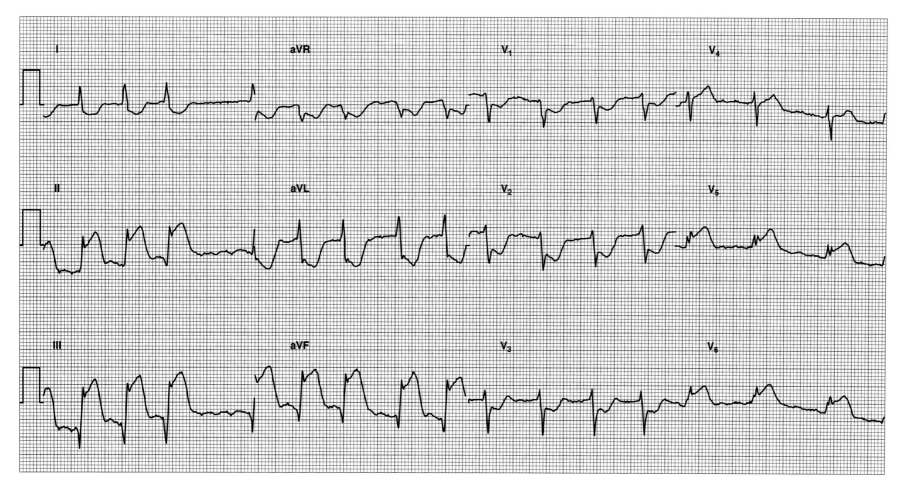

Rate and rhythm? _____ Pathologic Q waves? _____

STE? _____ ST depression? _____ T-wave changes? _____

Reciprocal changes? _____ STE variant present? _____ Axis? _____

Interpretation: _____

Inferior: II, III, aVF | Septum: V₁, V₂ | Anterior: V₃, V₄ | Lateral: I, aVL, V₅, V₆

Fig. **5.92**

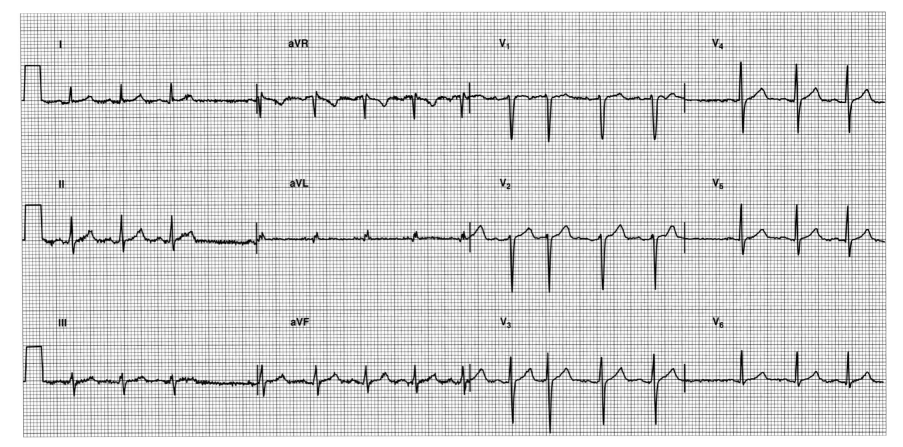

Rate and rhythm? _____ Pathologic Q waves? _____

STE? _____ ST depression? _____ T-wave changes? _____

Reciprocal changes? _____ STE variant present? _____ Axis? _____

Interpretation: _____

Inferior: II, III, aVF | Septum: V$_1$, V$_2$ | Anterior: V$_3$, V$_4$ | Lateral: I, aVL, V$_5$, V$_6$

Fig. **5.93**

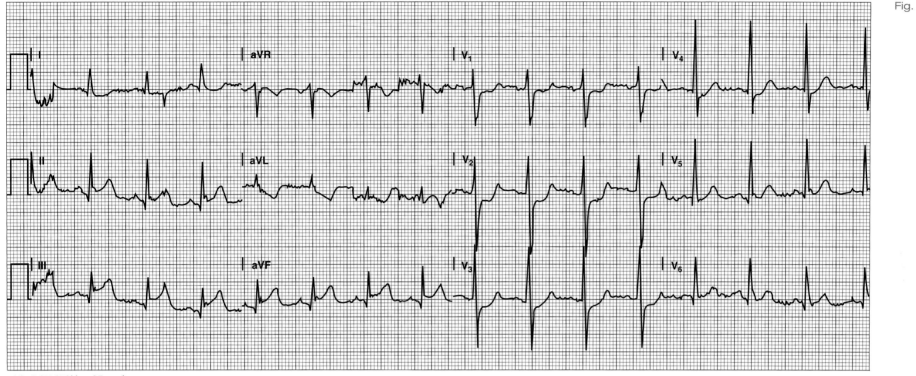

x1.0 0.05-150Hz   25mm/sec

Rate and rhythm? _____ Pathologic Q waves? _____

STE? _____ ST depression? _____ T-wave changes? _____

Reciprocal changes? _____ STE variant present? _____ Axis? _____

Interpretation: _____

Inferior: II, III, aVF | Septum: V₁, V₂ | Anterior: V₃, V₄ | **Lateral: I, aVL, V₅, V₆**

Fig. **5.94**

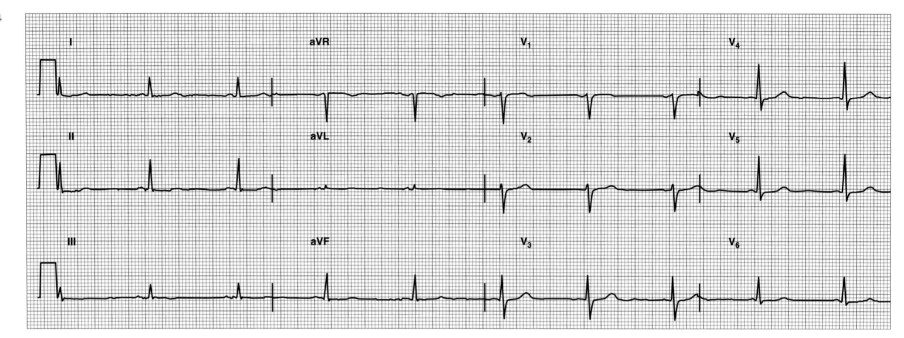

Rate and rhythm? _____ Pathologic Q waves? _____

STE? _____ ST depression? _____ T-wave changes? _____

Reciprocal changes? _____ STE variant present? _____ Axis? _____

Interpretation: _____

Inferior: II, III, aVF | **Septum: V₁, V₂** | **Anterior: V₃, V₄** | **Lateral: I, aVL, V₅, V₆**

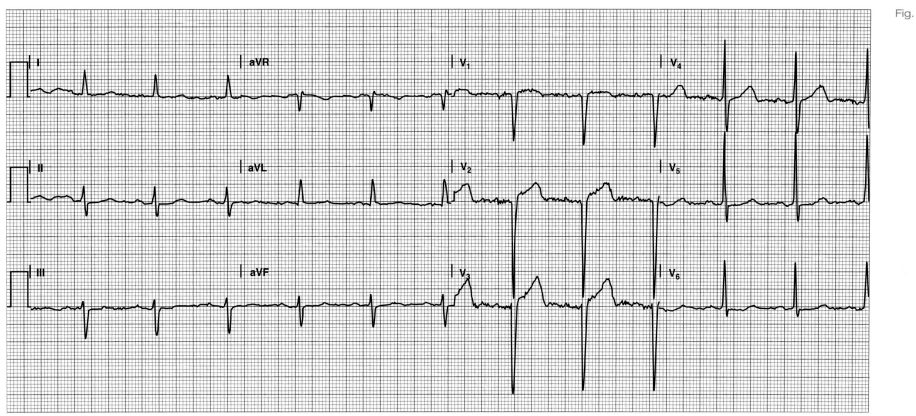

Fig. **5.95**

Rate and rhythm? _____ Pathologic Q waves? _____

STE? _____ ST depression? _____ T-wave changes? _____

Reciprocal changes? _____ STE variant present? _____ Axis? _____

Interpretation: _____

Inferior: II, III, aVF | Septum: V$_1$, V$_2$ | Anterior: V$_3$, V$_4$ | Lateral: I, aVL, V$_5$, V$_6$

Fig. 5.96

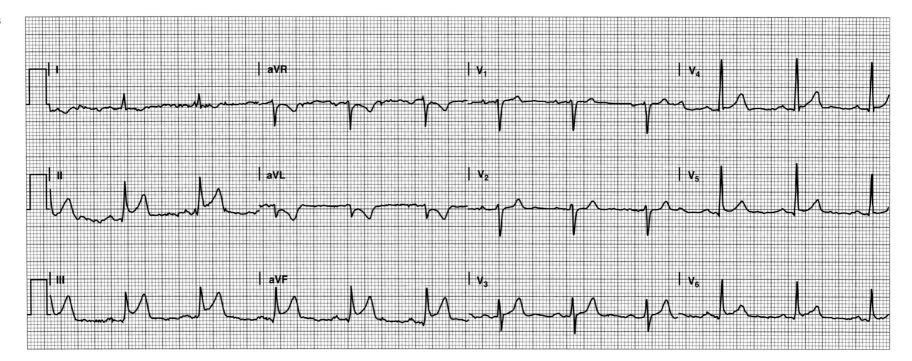

Rate and rhythm? _____ Pathologic Q waves? _____

STE? _____ ST depression? _____ T-wave changes? _____

Reciprocal changes? _____ STE variant present? _____ Axis? _____

Interpretation: _____

Inferior: II, III, aVF | Septum: V₁, V₂ | Anterior: V₃, V₄ | Lateral: I, aVL, V₅, V₆

Fig. **5.97**

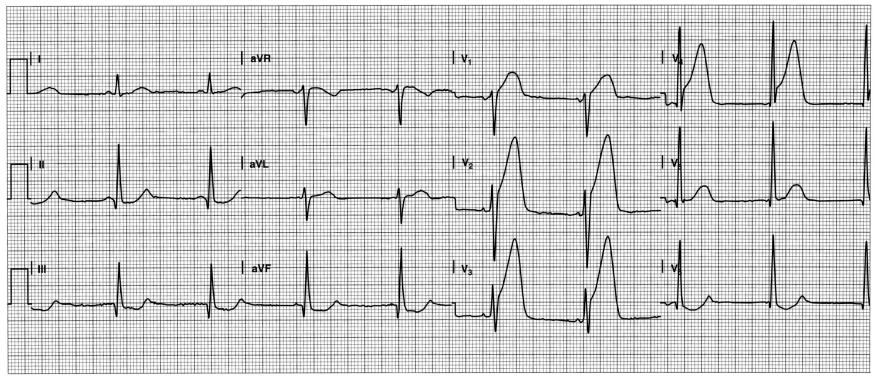

x1.0 0.05-150Hz   25mm/sec

Rate and rhythm? _____ Pathologic Q waves? _____

STE? _____ ST depression? _____ T-wave changes? _____

Reciprocal changes? _____ STE variant present? _____ Axis? _____

Interpretation: _____

Inferior: II, III, aVF | Septum: V₁, V₂ | Anterior: V₃, V₄ | **Lateral: I, aVL, V₅, V₆**

Fig. **5.98**

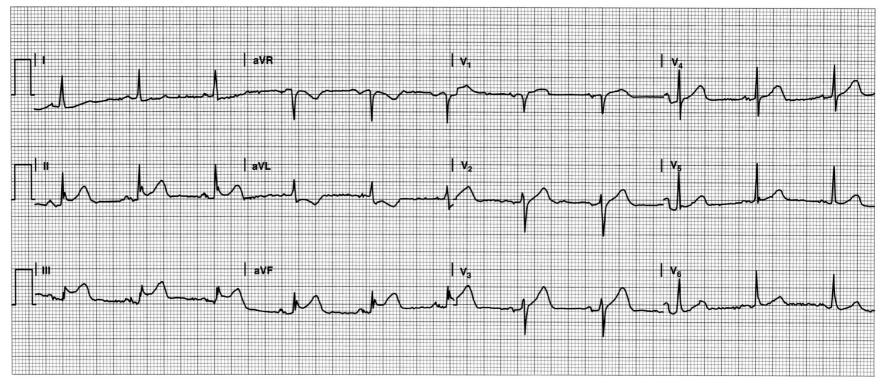

x1.0 0.05-150Hz 25mm/sec

Rate and rhythm? _____ Pathologic Q waves? _____

STE? _____ ST depression? _____ T-wave changes? _____

Reciprocal changes? _____ STE variant present? _____ Axis? _____

Interpretation: _____

Inferior: II, III, aVF | Septum: V₁, V₂ | Anterior: V₃, V₄ | Lateral: I, aVL, V₅, V₆

Fig. **5.99**

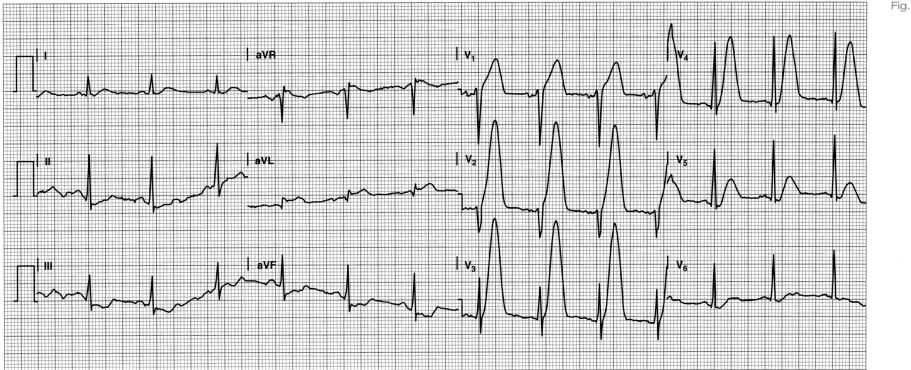

x1.0 0.05-150Hz 25mm/sec

Rate and rhythm? _____ Pathologic Q waves? _____

STE? _____ ST depression? _____ T-wave changes? _____

Reciprocal changes? _____ STE variant present? _____ Axis? _____

Interpretation: _____

Inferior: II, III, aVF | **Septum: V$_1$, V$_2$** | **Anterior: V$_3$, V$_4$** | **Lateral: I, aVL, V$_5$, V$_6$**

Fig. **5.100**

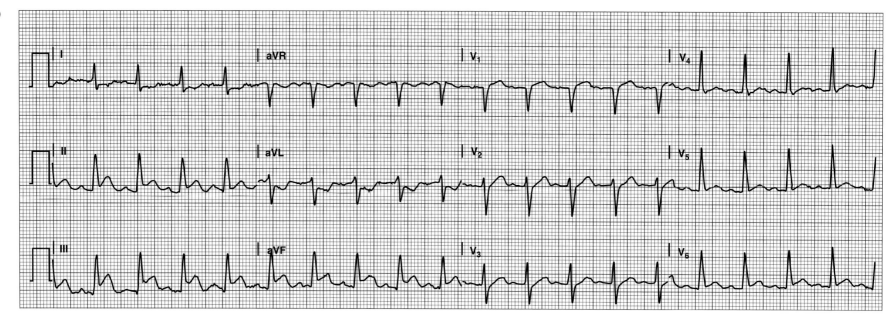

Rate and rhythm? _____ Pathologic Q waves? _____

STE? _____ ST depression? _____ T-wave changes? _____

Reciprocal changes? _____ STE variant present? _____ Axis? _____

Interpretation: _____

Inferior: II, III, aVF | Septum: V₁, V₂ | Anterior: V₃, V₄ | Lateral: I, aVL, V₅, V₆

INTERPRETATION OF PRACTICE ECGs

Fig. 5.1

Rate and rhythm:	Supraventricular bradycardia at 52 beats/min
STE:	II, III, aVF, V_3, V_5, V_6
ST depression:	aVL, V_1, V_2
T-wave changes:	Inverted in aVL, V_1, V_2
Reciprocal changes:	aVL
Axis:	Normal
Interpretation:	Inferolateral STEMI. Second-degree type I atrioventricular (AV) block present, probably nodal. ST depression and tall R wave in V_1 and V_2 suggest posterior wall involvement. Obtain right-sided chest leads to assess for right ventricular infarction (RVI), and posterior chest leads to assess for posterior MI. Note: STE in V_3 is probably due to the right coronary artery supplying a portion of the ventricular apex.

Fig. 5.2

Rate and rhythm:	Sinus rhythm at 90 beats/min
STE:	Slight in aVR and V_1
ST depression:	II, III, aVL, aVF, V_3 to V_6
Axis:	Normal
Interpretation:	Left bundle branch block (LBBB; QRS 112 msec). ST depression in eight or more leads plus slight STE in aVR and V_1 is associated with either three-vessel disease or a left main occlusion.

Fig. 5.3

Rate and rhythm:	Atrial fibrillation at 107 beats/min
ST depression:	V_6
T-wave changes:	Tall in V_2
Axis:	Normal
Interpretation:	Incomplete right bundle branch block (RBBB) pattern (RSR′ pattern in V_1 but QRS is within normal limits [90 msec]) Baseline wander in I and V_4 to V_6. Consider clinical presentation and use ST trending or serial ECGs.

Fig. 5.4

Rate and rhythm:	Sinus rhythm at 66 beats/min with first-degree AV block (PR interval 224 msec)
STE:	V_3
T-wave changes:	Inverted in aVL
STE variant present:	LVH
Axis:	Left
Interpretation:	LVH. Nonspecific intraventricular conduction delay (QRS 126 msec) with left axis deviation.

Fig. 5.5

Rate and rhythm:	Sinus tachycardia at 100 beats/min with ventricular demand pacemaker
Pathologic Q waves:	II, III, aVF, V_1 to V_4
STE:	V_1
ST depression:	I, aVL, V_5, V_6
STE variant present:	Ventricular-paced rhythm
Axis:	Left
Interpretation:	Ventricular-paced rhythm noted. Does not meet Sgarbossa criteria. Pacemaker can diminish STE that may otherwise be present. For that reason, consider STEMI. Consider clinical presentation and use ST trending or serial ECGs.

Fig. 5.6

Rate and rhythm:	Sinus bradycardia at 51 beats/min
Pathologic Q waves:	III, V_1
STE:	Slight in aVF, V_2
Axis:	Normal
Interpretation:	Sinus bradycardia. Low voltage in aVF; otherwise normal ECG.

Fig. 5.7

Rate and rhythm:	Sinus bradycardia at 51 beats/min
STE:	II, III, aVF
ST depression:	I, aVL, V$_1$ to V$_3$
T-wave changes:	Inverted in I, aVL, V$_1$ to V$_4$; tall in II, III, aVF
Reciprocal changes:	I, aVL
Axis:	Normal
Interpretation:	Inferior STEMI with nonspecific intraventricular conduction delay (QRS 112 msec). Reciprocal changes are present. ST depression in V$_1$ to V$_3$, possibly from posterior involvement (poor R-wave progression is present, but posterior STEMI often causes increased R-wave height). Consider obtaining posterior chest leads. Obtain V$_4$R to assess for RVI.

Fig. 5.8

Rate and rhythm:	Sinus rhythm at 71 beats/min
STE:	V$_1$ to V$_3$
ST depression:	II
T-wave changes:	Tall in V$_2$ to V$_4$
Axis:	Normal
Interpretation:	Possible anteroseptal STEMI (baseline wander makes it difficult to confirm).

Fig. 5.9

Rate and rhythm:	Sinus rhythm at 75 beats/min
Axis:	Left
Interpretation:	Low-voltage QRS complexes; poor R-wave progression; left axis deviation; baseline wander in V$_5$.

Fig. 5.10

Rate and rhythm:	Sinus rhythm at 95 beats/min
Pathologic Q waves:	I
STE:	aVL, V$_1$ to V$_4$
ST depression:	V$_5$?, V$_6$
T-wave changes:	Peaked in II, III, aVF; inverted in V$_2$ to V$_4$; not oppositely deflected from QRS in V$_5$, V$_6$
STE variant present:	LBBB
Axis:	Normal
Interpretation:	Anteroseptal STEMI with LBBB. In V$_4$, the J point is elevated and concordant with the QRS, which meets Sgarbossa criteria. Low-voltage QRS complexes in lead I. Baseline wander in I, II, III, aVL. Poor R-wave progression V$_2$ to V$_3$.

Fig. 5.11

Rate and rhythm:	Sinus tachycardia at 109 beats/min with occasional premature ventricular complexes (PVCs)
STE:	II, III, aVF
ST depression:	I, aVL, V$_2$
T-wave changes:	Inverted in I, aVL
Reciprocal changes:	I, aVL
Axis:	Normal
Interpretation:	Inferior STEMI with reciprocal changes. Obtain V$_4$R to assess for RVI. Because of the ST depression in V$_2$, consider obtaining posterior leads to assess for inferobasal infarction.

Fig. 5.12

Rate and rhythm:	Sinus rhythm at 60 beats/min
STE:	II, III, aVF
ST depression:	aVL
T-wave changes:	Tall/peaked in II, III, aVF, V$_3$ to V$_5$; inverted in aVL
Reciprocal changes:	aVL
Axis:	Normal
Interpretation:	Inferoapical infarct. Obtain V$_4$R to assess for RVI. Poor R-wave progression V$_2$ to V$_3$. Artifact I, II, III, aVL, aVF, V$_5$, V$_6$.

Fig. 5.13

Rate and rhythm:	Sinus arrhythmia at 62 beats/min with first-degree AV block (PR interval 262 msec)
T-wave changes:	Inverted in aVL, V_6
Axis:	Left
Interpretation:	Left anterior fascicular block (LAFB) (left axis deviation, qR pattern in aVL, QRS 116 msec). Low-voltage QRS complexes in V_2. Poor R-wave progression. Nonspecific T-wave abnormality.

Fig. 5.14

Rate and rhythm:	Sinus rhythm at 98 beats/min with LBBB
STE:	V_1 to V_4
STE variant present:	LBBB
Axis:	Left
Interpretation:	Possible anteroseptal STEMI versus new-onset LBBB (QRS 176 msec). The QRS amplitude is about 40 mV in V_2, and the STE is about 7 mm. The STE of 5 mm or more meets Sgarbossa criteria; however, recall that STE is the least persuasive of the Sgarbossa criteria. The STE would need to equal 10 mm or more to meet the modified Sgarbossa criteria. Therefore, this may be a new-onset LBBB. As always, consider clinical presentation and use ST trending or serial ECGs.

Fig. 5.15

Rate and rhythm:	Sinus rhythm at 82 beats/min
STE:	V_1 to V_3
STE variant present:	ER? Pericarditis?
Axis:	Normal
Interpretation:	Possible anteroseptal STEMI (STE noted in V_1 to V_3). ER and pericarditis are possible explanations for STE. In addition, slight STE in V_1 to V_3 can be a normal variant. Consider clinical presentation and use ST trending or serial ECGs.

Fig. 5.16

Rate and rhythm:	Sinus rhythm at 75 beats/min
STE:	V_2 and V_3
ST depression:	II, III, aVF
T-wave changes:	Tall in V_2 and V_3
Axis:	Normal
Interpretation:	Anteroseptal STEMI. STE and tall T waves are noted in V_2 and V_3. With tall T waves, hyperkalemia is a possibility, but in this case, the broad base of the T wave favors the hyperacute T wave of STEMI.

Fig. 5.17

Rate and rhythm:	Sinus rhythm at 85 beats/min
Pathologic Q waves:	V_1 to V_3
STE:	Slight in aVL, V_4
ST depression:	II, III, aVF
T-wave changes:	Inverted in II, III, aVF
Axis:	Right
Interpretation:	Slurring of the initial portion of the QRS (i.e., delta wave) seen in leads II, III, aVF, and V_6, and a wide QRS (114 msec) suggests the presence of Wolff-Parkinson-White (WPW) pattern. Consider clinical presentation (WPW vs. inferior ischemia). Poor R-wave progression.

Fig. 5.18

Rate and rhythm:	Atrial fibrillation at 81 beats/min
STE:	I, aVL
ST depression:	II, III, aVF
Reciprocal changes:	II, III, aVF
Axis:	Left
Interpretation:	High lateral STEMI. Reciprocal changes noted in II, III, and aVF.

Fig. 5.19

Rate and rhythm:	Electronic atrial pacemaker at 80 pulses/min
Axis:	Normal
Interpretation:	When the atria are paced with normal conduction in the ventricles, the typical rules for STE are still used. Consider clinical presentation and use ST trending or serial ECGs.

Fig. 5.20

Rate and rhythm:	Sinus rhythm at 85 beats/min
STE:	II, III, aVF
ST depression:	I, aVL, V_2 to V_6
T-wave changes:	Tall/peaked in II, III, aVF; inverted in aVL, V_1 to V_6
Reciprocal changes:	I, aVL
Axis:	Normal
Interpretation:	Inferior STEMI, reciprocal changes present. Possible posterior infarct (ST depression in septal and anterior chest leads). Poor R-wave progression in V_2 to V_6. Baseline wander and artifact in I and aVL. Obtain posterior and right-sided chest leads and consider clinical presentation.

Fig. 5.21

Rate and rhythm:	Atrial fibrillation with multiform PVCs; ventricular rate 82 to 117 beats/min
STE:	II, V_5
T-wave changes:	Inverted in aVL
Axis:	Left
Interpretation:	RBBB with LAFB (QRS 142 msec). Nearing criteria for LVH (patient is a 74-year-old Caucasian man).

Fig. 5.22

Rate and rhythm:	Sinus rhythm at 77 beats/min with first-degree AV block (PR interval 224 msec)
STE:	II, III, aVF
ST depression:	I, aVL, V_1, and V_2
T-wave changes:	Inverted in I, aVL, subtle in V_1, more prominent in V_2
Reciprocal changes:	I, aVL
Axis:	Normal
Interpretation:	Inferior STEMI, reciprocal changes present. Poor R-wave progression. Obtain right-sided chest leads and consider clinical presentation.

Fig. 5.23

Rate and rhythm:	Sinus rhythm at 71 beats/min with first-degree AV block (PR interval 212 msec)
Pathologic Q waves:	V_1 to V_3
STE:	V_2, V_3
ST depression:	V_5, V_6
Axis:	Left
Interpretation:	Possible anteroseptal STEMI. Poor R-wave progression. Artifact makes exact identification of the J point and TP segment difficult. QS complexes (counts as a pathologic Q wave) noted in V_1 to V_3. Consider STEMI versus normal variant versus previous acute MI with ventricular aneurysm. Consider clinical presentation and use ST trending or serial ECGs.

Fig. 5.24

Rate and rhythm:	Sinus rhythm at 91 beats/min with occasional PVCs
STE:	Slight in aVR
ST depression:	I, II, III, aVF, V_2 to V_6
Axis:	Normal
Interpretation:	Inferior and anterolateral ischemia. Because of the diffuse ST depression in multiple leads and slight STE in aVR, left main or three-vessel disease must be considered. Consider clinical presentation and use ST trending or serial ECGs.

Fig. 5.25

Rate and rhythm:	Sinus bradycardia at 59 beats/min
STE:	I, II, aVL, V_2 to V_6
ST depression:	III, aVR, aVF
T-wave changes:	Tall in V_2 to V_5
STE variant present:	Pericarditis?
Axis:	Normal
Interpretation:	Suspected global MI. Baseline wander in I, II, III. ECG quality makes interpretation difficult. Low-voltage QRS complexes in the limb leads. Lead V_1 looks mostly normal. If STE is due to STEMI, then the inferior, septal, anterior, and lateral walls are involved (more likely). If an STE variant, then pericarditis would be the only one to account for elevation in these leads (less likely). Consider clinical presentation and use ST trending or serial ECGs.

Fig. 5.26

Rate and rhythm:	Sinus rhythm at 73 beats/min with premature atrial complexes (PACs)
Axis:	Normal
Interpretation:	Normal ECG. Consider clinical presentation.

Fig. 5.27

Rate and rhythm:	Sinus rhythm at 94 beats/min
Pathologic Q waves:	III, aVF
STE:	II, III, aVF, V_1, V_3 to V_5
ST depression:	I, aVL
T-wave changes:	Tall in II, III, aVF; peaked in V_2
Reciprocal changes:	I, aVL
Axis:	Normal
Interpretation:	Inferior STEMI, reciprocal changes present. Possible RVI (STE greater in V_1 than V_2). Possible posterior infarction (tall R waves in early chest leads). Possible apical infarction (coving in V_3 and V_4). Artifact in lead I. Obtain posterior and right-sided chest leads and consider clinical presentation.

Fig. 5.28

Rate and rhythm:	Sinus rhythm at 67 beats/min
STE:	V_3
Axis:	Normal
Interpretation:	Incomplete RBBB (QRS 108 msec). This patient is a 16-year-old Caucasian boy who experienced a syncopal episode. Note the rSr′ with STE and an upright T wave in V_2, which creates a saddleback. This pattern may occur if electrodes are placed too high on the chest, it may be a normal variant, and it may be seen in patients with Brugada syndrome. Carefully consider the patient's history and clinical presentation.

Fig. 5.29

Rate and rhythm:	Sinus rhythm at 75 beats/min
STE:	V_2 to V_6
T-wave changes:	Inverted in V_1
Axis:	Left
Interpretation:	Anteroseptal STEMI with lateral extension. The artifact in I, II, III, and aVF makes it difficult to confirm whether STE exists in these leads.

Fig. 5.30

Rate and rhythm:	Sinus bradycardia at 54 beats/min
Pathologic Q waves:	II?, III? aVF?
STE:	II, III, aVF
ST depression:	I, aVL
T-wave changes:	Tall/peaked in III, aVF; flattened in V_5, V_6; inverted in I, aVL, V_2 to V_4
Reciprocal changes:	I, aVL
Axis:	Normal
Interpretation:	Inferior STEMI, reciprocal changes present. Possible posterior infarct. Possible previous anteroseptal infarct (poor R-wave progression V_2, V_3). Baseline wander in II, III, V_1, and V_6. Obtain posterior and right-sided chest leads and consider clinical presentation.

Fig. 5.31

Rate and rhythm:	Sinus rhythm at 74 beats/min with LBBB
Pathologic Q waves:	III, V_1, V_2
STE:	V_1 to V_3
ST depression:	V_6
T-wave changes:	Inverted in aVL, tall/peaked in V_2 to V_4
STE variant present:	LBBB
Axis:	Left
Interpretation:	LBBB (QRS 138 msec). Does not meet Sgarbossa criteria for infarct-induced LBBB. Consider clinical presentation and use ST trending or serial ECGs.

Fig. 5.32

Rate and rhythm:	Sinus bradycardia at 55 beats/min
STE:	V_5, V_6
T-wave changes:	Inverted in V_1
Axis:	Normal
Interpretation:	Borderline ST changes in V_5 and V_6. The shape of ST segment in II and aVF is suspicious as well. Consider clinical presentation and use ST trending or serial ECGs.

Fig. 5.33

Rate and rhythm:	Atrial flutter at 94 beats/min with variable AV block
ST depression:	V_5, V_6
T-wave changes:	Inverted in I, aVL, V_5, V_6
STE variant present:	LVH
Axis:	Left
Interpretation:	LVH (S in lead III + R in aVL = 21 mm) with repolarization abnormality. This patient is a 77-year-old Caucasian woman.

Fig. 5.34

Rate and rhythm:	Sinus rhythm at 78 beats/min with occasional ectopic premature complexes
STE:	V_1 to V_4
ST depression:	II, III, aVF
T-wave changes:	Tall/peaked in V_2 to V_5
Axis:	Normal
Interpretation:	Anteroseptal STEMI.

Fig. 5.35

Rate and rhythm:	Sinus tachycardia at 107 beats/min
T-wave changes:	Inverted in I, aVL; tall/peaked in V_2
Axis:	Normal
Interpretation:	Nonspecific T-wave abnormality. Artifact present in most leads. Consider clinical presentation.

Fig. 5.36

Rate and rhythm:	Sinus arrhythmia at 92 beats/min
STE:	II, III, aVF
ST depression:	I, aVL, V_2, V_4 to V_6
T-wave changes:	Tall in II, III, aVF; inverted in I, aVL, V_1, V_2
Reciprocal changes:	I, aVL
Axis:	Normal
Interpretation:	Inferior STEMI, reciprocal changes present. Obtain right-sided chest leads to assess for RVI and consider clinical presentation.

Fig. 5.37

Rate and rhythm:	Sinus rhythm at 75 beats/min with LBBB
STE:	V_1 to V_3
ST depression:	V_5, V_6
STE variant present:	LBBB
Axis:	Left
Interpretation:	Possible anteroseptal STEMI versus new-onset LBBB (QRS 144 msec). Does not meet Sgarbossa criteria for infarct-induced LBBB but cannot rule out that possibility. Consider clinical presentation and use ST trending or serial ECGs.

Fig. 5.38

Rate and rhythm:	Sinus rhythm at 83 beats/min with RBBB and LAFB
Pathologic Q waves:	I, aVL, V_3 to V_6
ST depression:	V_1 to V_4
T-wave changes:	Inverted in V_1 to V_4
Axis:	Left
Interpretation:	Bifascicular block (RBBB and LAFB). RBBB pattern (RSR' in V_1, QRS 152 msec); LAFB (left axis deviation, QR pattern in aVL). Consider clinical presentation.

Fig. 5.39

Rate and rhythm:	Sinus rhythm at 62 beats/min
STE:	I, aVL, V_2 to V_6
ST depression:	III, aVF
T-wave changes:	Tall in V_2 to V_5
Reciprocal changes:	III, aVF
Axis:	Left
Interpretation:	Extensive anterolateral STEMI, reciprocal changes present. Consider clinical presentation and use ST trending or serial ECGs.

Fig. 5.40

Rate and rhythm:	Sinus arrhythmia at 61 beats/min with LBBB
STE:	V_1, V_2
ST depression:	V_4 to V_6
T-wave changes:	Inverted in I, aVL
STE variant present:	LBBB
Axis:	Left
Interpretation:	LBBB pattern present (QRS 142 msec). Consider clinical presentation and use ST trending or serial ECGs.

Fig. 5.41

Rate and rhythm:	Sinus rhythm at 95 beats/min
Pathologic Q waves:	V_2
STE:	V_1 to V_3
T-wave changes:	Inverted in aVL
Axis:	Left
Interpretation:	Anteroseptal STEMI (if clinical picture suggests acute MI). Baseline wander in V_5 and V_6. STE in V_1 to V_3 and T-wave inversion suggest possible STEMI. However, the QS complex in V_2 and poor R-wave progression through V_4 make previous MI with persistent STE a distinct possibility. Consider clinical presentation and use ST trending or serial ECGs.

Fig. 5.42

Rate and rhythm:	Sinus rhythm at 91 beats/min
Pathologic Q waves:	III, aVF
Axis:	Left
Interpretation:	QS complexes noted in III and aVF, possible previous inferior MI. Consider clinical presentation.

Fig. 5.43

Rate and rhythm:	Sinus rhythm at 79 beats/min
STE:	V_2 to V_6
T-wave changes:	Inverted in III, V_1
STE variant present:	ER?
Axis:	Normal
Interpretation:	Artifact in V_1. Probable J-point elevation of 1 mm in V_2. STE in V_3 to V_6. This patient is a 33-year-old Caucasian man. ER is a possible cause of STE (STE with normally inflected T wave). Consider clinical presentation.

Fig. 5.44

Rate and rhythm:	Sinus bradycardia at 58 beats/min
STE:	V_1 to V_3
ST depression:	III, aVF
T-wave changes:	Inverted in III, tall in V_2 to V_4
Axis:	Left
Interpretation:	Anteroseptal STEMI. Consider clinical presentation and use ST trending or serial ECGs.

Fig. 5.45

Rate and rhythm:	Sinus rhythm at 65 beats/min
STE:	II, III, aVF
ST depression:	I, aVL
T-wave changes:	Tall/peaked in II, III, aVF, V_3 to V_6; inverted in I, aVL
Reciprocal changes:	I, aVL
Axis:	Normal
Interpretation:	Inferior STEMI, reciprocal changes present. Obtain right-sided chest leads to assess for RVI and consider clinical presentation.

Fig. 5.46

Rate and rhythm:	Sinus rhythm at 68 beats/min
Pathologic Q waves:	III, aVF
STE:	II, III, aVF, V_5, V_6
ST depression:	I, aVL, V_1 to V_4
T-wave changes:	Tall/peaked in II, III, aVF; inverted in I, aVL, V_2, V_3
Reciprocal changes:	I, aVL
Axis:	Normal
Interpretation:	Inferolateral STEMI, reciprocal changes present. Possible posterior infarct (ST depression V_1 to V_4). Poor R-wave progression in V_4 and V_5. Artifact in I and II. Obtain posterior and right-sided chest leads and consider clinical presentation.

Fig. 5.47

Rate and rhythm:	Sinus rhythm at 75 beats/min
Axis:	Normal
Interpretation:	Normal ECG. Artifact in V_1.

Fig. 5.48

Rate and rhythm:	Sinus rhythm at 76 beats/min with LBBB
STE:	V_1 to V_4
T-wave changes:	Inverted in I, aVL, V_5, V_6
STE variant present:	LBBB
Axis:	Left
Interpretation:	Possible anteroseptal STEMI versus new-onset LBBB (QRS 144 msec). Does not meet Sgarbossa criteria for infarct-induced LBBB but cannot rule out that possibility. Consider clinical presentation and use ST trending or serial ECGs.

Fig. 5.49

Rate and rhythm:	Sinus tachycardia at 136 beats/min with short PR interval (116 msec), short QT interval (228 msec)
STE:	Borderline in II, III, aVF
ST depression:	aVL
T-wave changes:	Inverted in aVL
Reciprocal changes:	aVL
STE variant present:	Pericarditis?
Axis:	Normal
Interpretation:	Possible inferior STEMI. Artifact makes J point and baseline determination difficult. ECG is not typical for ER, but pericarditis is a consideration given the less-than-obvious reciprocal changes in aVL and PR-segment elevation in aVR. Obtain right-sided chest leads to assess for RVI, consider clinical presentation, and use ST trending or serial ECGs.

Fig. 5.50

Rate and rhythm:	Sinus rhythm at 83 beats/min with first-degree AV block and RBBB (PR interval 228 msec, QRS 156 msec)
STE:	III, aVF
ST depression:	I, aVL, V_3 to V_6
T-wave changes:	Inverted in I, V_1, V_4 to V_6
Reciprocal changes:	I, aVL
Axis:	Right
Interpretation:	Possible inferior STEMI versus RBBB. STE noted in III and minimal amount in aVF. RBBB pattern noted. RBBB can cause STE. The concordant STE in III suggests STEMI. Obtain right-sided chest leads, consider clinical presentation, and use ST trending or serial ECGs.

Fig. 5.51

Rate and rhythm:	Sinus arrhythmia at 67 beats/min
T-wave changes:	Inverted in V_1
Axis:	Normal
Interpretation:	Normal ECG; ST depression is present in one complex in lead III but not in the others.

Fig. 5.52

Rate and rhythm:	Sinus rhythm at 61 beats/min with occasional premature supraventricular beats
STE:	II, III; slight in V_5, V_6
ST depression:	I, aVL, V_1, V_2
T-wave changes:	Inverted in I, aVL, V_1, V_2
Reciprocal changes:	I, aVL
Axis:	Normal
Interpretation:	Inferior STEMI; reciprocal changes present. Obtain right-sided chest leads, consider clinical presentation, and use ST trending or serial ECGs.

Fig. 5.53

Rate and rhythm:	Atrial fibrillation at 153 beats/min with a premature aberrantly conducted complex
ST depression:	I, II, aVL, V_6
Axis:	Left
Interpretation:	Nonspecific ST abnormality. Consider clinical presentation and use ST trending or serial ECGs.

Fig. 5.54

Rate and rhythm:	Sinus rhythm at 86 beats/min
STE:	V_2 to V_5
T-wave changes:	Tall in V_2 to V_5; inverted in III
STE variant present:	ER?
Axis:	Normal
Interpretation:	Possible anteroseptal STEMI versus ER. Probably ER (STE with normally inflected T wave). This patient is a 21-year-old Caucasian man. Consider clinical presentation and use ST trending or serial ECGs.

Fig. 5.55

Rate and rhythm:	Wide QRS tachycardia at 181 beats/min (QRS 252 msec)
STE variant present:	Ventricular rhythm; LBBB
Axis:	Left
Interpretation:	Wide QRS tachycardia (probably atrial fibrillation with LBBB). Both supraventricular tachycardia (SVT) with aberrant conduction and ventricular tachycardia (VT) can produce STE. Consider clinical presentation and use ST trending or serial ECGs.

Fig. 5.56

Rate and rhythm:	Junctional rhythm at 55 beats/min
STE:	II, III, aVF
ST depression:	I, aVL, V_1 to V_4
T-wave changes:	Inverted in aVL, V_1
Reciprocal changes:	aVL
Axis:	Normal
Interpretation:	Inferior STEMI; probable posterior MI as well. Obtain right-sided and posterior chest leads and consider clinical presentation.

Fig. 5.57

Rate and rhythm:	Sinus rhythm at 93 beats/min
STE:	II, III, aVF, V_4 to V_6
ST depression:	aVL, V_1 to V_3
T-wave changes:	Inverted in V_1, V_2
Reciprocal changes:	aVL
Axis:	Normal
Interpretation:	Inferolateral STEMI. ST depression in V_1 to V_3 suggestive of posterior wall involvement. Obtain right-sided and posterior chest leads and consider clinical presentation.

Fig. 5.58

Rate and rhythm:	Sinus tachycardia at 153 beats/min with LAFB
Pathologic Q waves:	II, V_1 to V_3
STE:	III, aVF, V_3, V_4
ST depression:	aVL, V_5, V_6
T-wave changes:	Inverted in V_5, V_6
Reciprocal changes:	aVL
Axis:	Left
Interpretation:	Possible inferior STEMI, LAFB. Anteroseptal infarct, age undetermined. Artifact in most leads. Approaching criteria for LVH. Obtain right-sided chest leads, consider clinical presentation, and use ST trending or serial ECGs.

Fig. 5.59

Rate and rhythm:	Sinus rhythm at 73 beats/min with LBBB
STE:	V_1, V_2
ST depression:	I, II, aVL, aVF, V_5, V_6
STE variant present:	LBBB
Axis:	Left
Interpretation:	Possible septal STEMI versus new-onset LBBB (QRS 144 msec). Does not meet Sgarbossa criteria for infarct-induced LBBB but cannot rule out that possibility. Consider clinical presentation and use ST trending or serial ECGs.

Fig. 5.60

Rate and rhythm:	Sinus rhythm at 74 beats/min
STE:	V_5, V_6
T-wave changes:	Inverted in aVL
Axis:	Normal
Interpretation:	Possible lateral STEMI. STE of 1 mm in V_6 but borderline in V_5. ECG quality makes it difficult to be certain about V_5. Consider clinical presentation and use ST trending or serial ECGs.

Fig. 5.61

Rate and rhythm:	Ventricular-paced rhythm at 91 pulses/min
STE:	II, III, aVF
ST depression:	I, aVL, V_2 to V_4
T-wave changes:	Tall in II, III, aVF; inverted in I, aVL
Reciprocal changes:	I, aVL
STE variant present:	Ventricular-paced rhythm
Axis:	Left
Interpretation:	Possible inferior STEMI. Wide QRS (164 msec) and ventricular pacemaker noted. A ventricular pacemaker can account for STE; however, a paced rhythm does not rule out STEMI. With a paced rhythm, 5 mm or more of STE suggests STEMI. In leads II and III, that criteria may be met. A steadier baseline would add more certainty to the measurement. The concordant ST depression is also suggestive of STEMI. Obtain right-sided chest leads, consider clinical presentation, and use ST trending or serial ECGs.

Fig. 5.62

Rate and rhythm:	Sinus rhythm at 89 beats/min
Axis:	Normal
Interpretation:	Nonspecific T-wave abnormality; baseline wander in V_5 and V_6. Artifact in most limb leads. Consider clinical presentation.

Fig. 5.63

Rate and rhythm:	Sinus rhythm at 82 beats/min
STE:	V_1 to V_3
T-wave changes:	Inverted in III, tall in V_2, V_3
Axis:	Normal
Interpretation:	Borderline STE in V_1 to V_3, especially in V_2. Close but does not appear to meet STE criteria at this time. Consider clinical presentation and use ST trending or serial ECGs.

Fig. 5.64

Rate and rhythm:	Sinus rhythm at 99 beats/min
STE:	aVR
ST depression:	I, II, aVL, V_4 to V_6
Axis:	Normal
Interpretation:	Widespread ST depression noted. Baseline wander in I and III. Artifact in most limb leads. Consider clinical presentation.

Fig. 5.65

Rate and rhythm:	Sinus bradycardia at 58 beats/min
STE:	I, aVL, V_2 to V_6
ST depression:	II, III, aVF
Reciprocal changes:	II, III, aVF
Axis:	Normal
Interpretation:	Extensive anterolateral STEMI. Consider clinical presentation and use ST trending or serial ECGs.

Fig. 5.66

Rate and rhythm:	Sinus bradycardia at 56 beats/min
T-wave changes:	Inverted in V_1
Axis:	Normal
Interpretation:	Sinus bradycardia, otherwise normal ECG. Consider clinical presentation.

Fig. 5.67

Rate and rhythm:	Sinus rhythm at 71 beats/min
STE:	II, III, aVF
ST depression:	V_2 to V_4
T-wave changes:	Inverted in V_1
Reciprocal changes:	aVL
Axis:	Normal
Interpretation:	Inferior STEMI. Low QRS voltage in limb leads. ST depression in V_2 to V_4 suggestive of posterior wall involvement. Obtain right-sided and posterior chest leads and consider clinical presentation.

Fig. 5.68

Rate and rhythm:	Sinus rhythm at 60 beats/min with LBBB
STE:	V_1 to V_4
ST depression:	I, aVL, V_5, V_6
T-wave changes:	Inverted in I, aVL, V_5, V_6
STE variant present:	LBBB
Axis:	Left
Interpretation:	Possible anteroseptal STEMI versus new-onset LBBB (QRS 136 msec). Does not meet Sgarbossa criteria for infarct-induced LBBB but cannot rule out that possibility. Consider clinical presentation and use ST trending or serial ECGs.

Fig. 5.69

Rate and rhythm:	Sinus rhythm at 74 beats/min with RBBB
Pathologic Q waves:	III, aVF
T-wave changes:	Inverted in V_1, V_2
Axis:	Left
Interpretation:	RBBB pattern noted (QRS 130 msec). While no ECG evidence exists to suspect STEMI, the RBBB can diminish STE that might otherwise be present. Consider clinical presentation. Artifact in limb leads and V_1; baseline wander in V_1 and V_2.

Fig. 5.70

Rate and rhythm:	Sinus rhythm at 86 beats/min
STE:	V_1 to V_4
T-wave changes:	Inverted in III; tall/peaked in V_2 to V_4
Axis:	Normal
Interpretation:	Anteroseptal STEMI. Baseline wander in V_6. Consider clinical presentation and use ST trending or serial ECGs.

Fig. 5.71

Rate and rhythm:	Sinus rhythm at 74 beats/min
T-wave changes:	Tall in V_1 to V_4
Axis:	Normal
Interpretation:	Although this ECG does not meet the STE criteria for STEMI, there are tall T waves in V_1 to V_4, which makes it very possible that this is the hyperacute phase of a STEMI. Consider clinical presentation and use ST trending or serial ECGs.

Fig. 5.72

Rate and rhythm:	Atrial fibrillation at 87 beats/min with RBBB
Axis:	Right
Interpretation:	RBBB pattern present (QRS 136 msec). RVH present (tall R waves in V_1, deeper-than-normal S waves in V_5 and V_6). Consider clinical presentation.

Fig. 5.73

Rate and rhythm:	Sinus rhythm at 78 beats/min
Pathologic Q waves:	II, III, aVF
STE:	I, aVL, V_2 to V_5
ST depression:	II, III, aVF
T-wave changes:	Inverted in II, III, aVF
Reciprocal changes:	II, III, aVF
Axis:	Left
Interpretation:	Suspected extensive anterolateral STEMI. RSR (QR) in V_1/V_2 is consistent with right ventricular conduction delay (QRS 128 msec). Consider clinical presentation and use ST trending or serial ECGs.

Fig. 5.74

Rate and rhythm:	Sinus rhythm at 95 beats/min
ST depression:	V_2 to V_5
T-wave changes:	Inverted in III
Axis:	Normal
Interpretation:	Consider isolated posterior infarction; obtain additional leads. Nonspecific intraventricular conduction delay (QRS 112 msec). Consider clinical presentation.

Fig. 5.75

Rate and rhythm:	Supraventricular bradycardia at 42 beats/min
STE:	II, III, aVF, V_2 to V_6
ST depression:	I, aVL
Reciprocal changes:	I, aVL
Axis:	Normal
Interpretation:	Inferolateral STEMI with reciprocal changes. Baseline wander in the limb leads. Obtain right-sided chest leads. Consider clinical presentation and use ST trending or serial ECGs.

Fig. 5.76

Rate and rhythm:	Sinus tachycardia at 140 beats/min with occasional ectopic premature complexes and LBBB
STE:	I, aVL, V_4 to V_6
ST depression:	II, III, aVF
Reciprocal changes:	II, III, aVF
STE variant present:	LBBB
Axis:	Left
Interpretation:	Lateral STEMI, concordant STE in V_4 to V_6 in the presence of LBBB (QRS 124 msec). Meets Sgarbossa criteria (concordant STE in at least one lead). Possible left atrial enlargement. Looking at the discernible P waves, it is possible that atrial flutter is present and another flutter wave is not being conducted, which could cause an alteration of the J point. However, we believe that despite this possibility, genuine STE exists in V_4 and V_5 and in I and aVL (just not as clear-cut). Baseline wander in most leads. Consider clinical presentation and use ST trending or serial ECGs.

Fig. 5.77

Rate and rhythm:	Sinus bradycardia at 55 beats/min
STE:	II, III, aVF, V_2 to V_6
ST depression:	aVL
T-wave changes:	Tall in II, aVF, V_2 to V_4
Reciprocal changes:	aVL
STE variant present:	Pericarditis?
Axis:	Normal
Interpretation:	Global STEMI. With such widespread STE, pericarditis is a consideration. However, the ST depression in aVL (the lead most likely to show a reciprocal change with inferior STEMI) suggests STEMI. Artifact present in most limb leads; baseline wander in most chest leads. Consider clinical presentation and use ST trending or serial ECGs.

Fig. 5.78

Rate and rhythm:	Sinus bradycardia at 54 beats/min
STE:	V_1 to V_4
T-wave changes:	Inverted in I, aVL, V_6
STE variant present:	LBBB
Axis:	Normal
Interpretation:	LBBB (QRS 160 msec) STE in the presence of LBBB is generally seen in leads V_1 to V_3 but sometimes extends to V_4 and beyond. This ECG demonstrates this pattern. Artifact present in III, aVL, and V_4 to V_6. Consider clinical presentation.

Fig. 5.79

Rate and rhythm:	Sinus tachycardia at 136 beats/min
Pathologic Q waves:	V_1 to V_4
Axis:	Normal
Interpretation:	Low-voltage QRS. Baseline wander in I, III, and V_6. Consider clinical presentation.

Fig. 5.80

Rate and rhythm:	Sinus bradycardia at 50 beats/min with short (104 msec) PR interval
ST depression:	II, III, aVF, V_4 to V_6
T-wave changes:	Biphasic in V_3, inverted in V_4 to V_6
Axis:	Right
Interpretation:	Anterolateral ischemia. Consider clinical presentation and use ST trending or serial ECGs.

Fig. 5.81

Rate and rhythm:	Sinus rhythm at 78 beats/min with first-degree AV block (PR interval 220 msec)
STE:	V_2
ST depression:	I, aVL, V_4 to V_6
T-wave changes:	Inverted in I, aVL, V_4 to V_6
STE variant present:	LVH
Axis:	Left
Interpretation:	Possible lateral ischemia. Criteria met for LVH. Consider clinical presentation and use ST trending or serial ECGs.

Fig. 5.82

Rate and rhythm:	Sinus rhythm at 81 beats/min
Pathologic Q waves:	V_1, V_2
STE:	V_1 to V_4
ST depression:	II, III, aVF
T-wave changes:	Tall in V_2 to V_4
Axis:	Normal
Interpretation:	Anteroseptal STEMI. Consider clinical presentation and use ST trending or serial ECGs.

Fig. 5.83

Rate and rhythm:	Sinus arrhythmia at 64 beats/min
STE:	II, aVF, V_5, V_6
ST depression:	V_2
T-wave changes:	Inverted in V_1
STE variant present:	Pericarditis?
Axis:	Normal
Interpretation:	Inferolateral STEMI. No obvious reciprocal changes are noted, so pericarditis is possible but unlikely because of localized elevation. Obtain right-sided chest leads. Consider clinical presentation and use ST trending or serial ECGs.

Fig. 5.84

Rate and rhythm:	Sinus rhythm at 73 beats/min
Pathologic Q waves:	V_2, V_4
STE:	I, aVL, V_1 to V_5
ST depression:	II, III, aVF
T-wave changes:	Tall in V_2 to V_5
Reciprocal changes	II, III, aVF
Axis:	Normal
Interpretation:	Extensive anterolateral STEMI. Consider clinical presentation and use ST trending or serial ECGs.

Fig. 5.85

Rate and rhythm:	Supraventricular rhythm at 91 beats/min
STE:	V_1 to V_3
ST depression:	I, II, aVL, V_4 to V_6
T-wave changes:	Inverted in I, aVL, V_4 to V_6
STE variant present:	LVH
Axis:	Left
Interpretation:	Poor ECG quality. Possible anteroseptal STEMI. Voltage criteria for LVH met. Consider clinical presentation and use ST trending or serial ECGs.

Fig. 5.86

Rate and rhythm:	Sinus rhythm at 100 beats/min
Pathologic Q waves:	III
STE:	III, aVF; borderline in II
ST depression:	aVL
T-wave changes:	aVL
Reciprocal changes:	aVL
Axis:	Normal
Interpretation:	Inferior STEMI with reciprocal changes. Obtain right-sided chest leads, consider clinical presentation, and use ST trending or serial ECGs.

Fig. 5.87

Rate and rhythm:	Sinus rhythm at 69 beats/min with occasional premature complexes
T-wave changes:	Tall in V_4, V_5
Axis:	Normal
Interpretation:	RSR′ (QR) in V_1/V_2 is consistent with right ventricular conduction delay (QRS 110 msec). Consider clinical presentation.

Fig. 5.88

Rate and rhythm:	Sinus tachycardia at 113 beats/min with first-degree AV block (PR interval 332 msec) and LBBB
STE:	V_1 to V_3
ST depression:	V_6
STE variant present:	LBBB
Axis:	Normal
Interpretation:	Possible anteroseptal STEMI; however, wide QRS (146 msec) and LBBB pattern are also present. Artifact in limb leads. Consider clinical presentation and use ST trending or serial ECGs.

Fig. 5.89

Rate and rhythm:	Sinus tachycardia at 107 beats/min
STE:	II, III, aVF
ST depression:	I, aVL
T-wave changes:	Inverted in I, aVL
Reciprocal changes:	I, aVL
Axis:	Normal
Interpretation:	Inferior STEMI with reciprocal changes. Obtain right-sided chest leads, consider clinical presentation, and use ST trending or serial ECGs.

Fig. 5.90

Rate and rhythm:	Sinus rhythm at 84 beats/min
Axis:	Normal
Interpretation:	Normal ECG. Consider clinical presentation.

Fig. 5.91

Rate and rhythm:	Atrial fibrillation at 115 beats/min
Pathologic Q waves:	III, aVF
STE:	II, III, aVF, V_5, V_6
ST depression:	I, aVL, aVF, V_1 to V_3
T-wave changes:	Inverted in V_1, V_2
Reciprocal changes:	I, aVL
Axis:	Right
Interpretation:	Inferolateral STEMI with reciprocal changes. ST depression in V_1 to V_3 suggests possible posterior involvement. Obtain right-sided and posterior chest leads, consider clinical presentation, and use ST trending or serial ECGs.

Fig. 5.92

Rate and rhythm:	Sinus rhythm at 92 beats/min with nonconducted PACs
Axis:	Normal
Interpretation:	Sinus rhythm with nonconducted PACs; otherwise, normal ECG. Artifact present in the limb leads. Consider clinical presentation.

Fig. 5.93

Rate and rhythm:	Sinus rhythm at 92 beats/min
Pathologic Q waves:	II, III, aVF
STE:	II, III, aVF
ST depression:	I, aVL, V_1 to V_4
Reciprocal changes:	I, aVL
Axis:	Normal
Interpretation:	Inferior STEMI with reciprocal changes. ST depression in V_1 to V_4 suggests possible posterior involvement. Baseline wander in I, II, and III. Obtain right-sided and posterior chest leads, consider clinical presentation, and use ST trending or serial ECGs.

Fig. 5.94

Rate and rhythm:	Sinus rhythm at 84 beats/min
Axis:	Normal
Interpretation:	Normal ECG. Consider clinical presentation.

Fig. 5.95

Rate and rhythm:	Sinus rhythm at 71 beats/min with first-degree AV block (PR interval 212 msec)
Pathologic Q waves:	V_1, V_2
STE:	V_2, V_3
Axis:	Left
Interpretation:	Anteroseptal STEMI. Meets STE criteria in V_2 and V_3. Poor R-wave progression noted through V_3. Slight STE may be a normal variant in the range of V_1 to V_3. Borderline criteria for LVH. Although STEMI ECG criteria are met, integrating the clinical picture is particularly important with this ECG. Use ST trending or serial ECGs.

Fig. 5.96

Rate and rhythm:	Sinus rhythm at 69 beats/min
STE:	II, III, aVF
ST depression:	aVL
T-wave changes:	Inverted in I, aVL
Reciprocal changes:	I, aVL
Axis:	Normal
Interpretation:	Inferior STEMI with reciprocal changes. Obtain right-sided chest leads, consider clinical presentation, and use ST trending or serial ECGs.

Fig. 5.97

Rate and rhythm:	Sinus bradycardia at 56 beats/min with short (116 msec) PR interval
STE:	V_1 to V_4
ST depression:	II, III, aVF
T-wave changes:	Tall in V_2 to V_4
Axis:	Normal
Interpretation:	Anteroseptal STEMI. Consider clinical presentation and use ST trending or serial ECGs.

Fig. 5.98

Rate and rhythm:	Sinus rhythm at 65 beats/min
STE:	II, III, aVF
ST depression:	aVL
T-wave changes:	Inverted in aVL
Reciprocal changes:	aVL
Axis:	Normal
Interpretation:	Inferior STEMI with reciprocal changes. Baseline wander in I and III. Obtain right-sided chest leads, consider clinical presentation, and use ST trending or serial ECGs.

Fig. 5.99

Rate and rhythm:	Sinus rhythm at 81 beats/min
STE:	aVL, V_1 to V_2
ST depression:	II, III, aVF
T-wave changes:	Inverted in III; tall/peaked in V_1 to V_4
Axis:	Normal
Interpretation:	Septal STEMI. STE noted in V_1 to V_2 (aVL suspicious, but ECG quality makes it difficult to be certain). Baseline wander in most limb leads. Consider clinical presentation and use ST trending or serial ECGs.

Fig. 5.100

Rate and rhythm:	Sinus tachycardia at 114 beats/min
STE:	II, III, aVF
ST depression:	I, aVL
Reciprocal changes:	I, aVL
Axis:	Normal
Interpretation:	Inferior STEMI with reciprocal changes. Subtle ST changes are noted in V_5 and V_6 but do not meet criteria. Artifact present in I and III. Obtain right-sided chest leads, consider clinical presentation, and use ST trending or serial ECGs.

Index

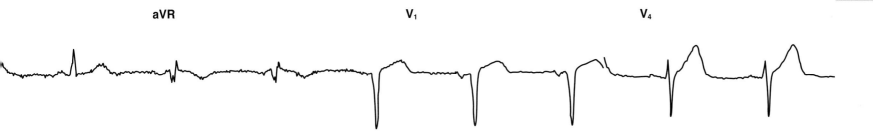

aVR   V₁   V₄

Note: Page numbers followed by *f* indicate figures, *t* indicates tables, and *b* indicate boxes.